Fieldwork for Healthcare:

Case Studies Investigating Human Factors in Computing Systems

Synthesis Lectures on Assistive, Rehabilitative, and Health-Preserving Technologies

Editor
Ron Baecker, *University of Toronto*

Advances in medicine allow us to live longer, despite the assaults on our bodies from war, environmental damage, and natural disasters. The result is that many of us survive for years or decades with increasing difficulties in tasks such as seeing, hearing, moving, planning, remembering, and communicating.

This series provides current state-of-the-art overviews of key topics in the burgeoning field of assistive technologies. We take a broad view of this field, giving attention not only to prosthetics that compensate for impaired capabilities, but to methods for rehabilitating or restoring function, as well as protective interventions that enable individuals to be healthy for longer periods of time throughout the lifespan. Our emphasis is in the role of information and communications technologies in prosthetics, rehabilitation, and disease prevention.

Fieldwork for Healthcare: Case Studies Investigating Human Factors in Computing Systems
Dominic Furniss, Aisling Ann O'Kane, Rebecca Randell, Svetlena Taneva, Helena Mentis, and Ann Blandford
2014

Interactive Technologies for Autism
Julie A. Kientz, Matthew S. Goodwin, Gillian R. Hayes, Gregory D. Abowd
2013

Patient-Centered Design of Cognitive Assistive Technology for Traumatic Brain Injury Telerehabilitation
Elliot Cole
2013

Zero Effort Technologies: Considerations, Challenges, and Use in Health, Wellness, and Rehabilitation
Alex Mihailidis, Jennifer Boger, Jesse Hoey, and Tizneem Jiancaro
2011

Design and the Digital Divide: Insights from 40 Years in Computer Support for Older and Disabled People
Alan F. Newell
2011

Fieldwork for Healthcare: Case Studies Investigating Human Factors in Computing Systems
Editors: Dominic Furniss, Aisling Ann O'Kane, Rebecca Randell, Svetlena Taneva, Helena Mentis, and Ann Blandford
www.morganclaypool.com

ISBN: 9781627053198 print
ISBN: 9781627053204 ebook

DOI 10.2200/S00552ED1V01Y201311ARH005

A Publication in the Morgan & Claypool Publishers series
SYNTHESIS LECTURES ON ASSISTIVE, REHABILITATIVE, AND HEALTH-PRESERVING TECHNOLOGIES #5
Series Editor: Ronald M. Baecker, University of Toronto

Series ISSN 2162-7258 Print   2162-7266 Electronic

Fieldwork for Healthcare:

Case Studies Investigating Human Factors in Computing Systems

Dominic Furniss
UCL Interaction Centre, University College London
Aisling Ann O'Kane
UCL Interaction Centre, University College London
Rebecca Randell
School of Healthcare, University of Leeds
Svetlena Taneva
Healthcare Human Factors, University Health Network, Toronto
Helena Mentis
Department of Information Systems, University of Maryland, Baltimore County
Ann Blandford
UCL Interaction Centre, University College London

SYNTHESIS LECTURES ON ASSISTIVE, REHABILITATIVE, AND HEALTH-PRESERVING TECHNOLOGIES # 5

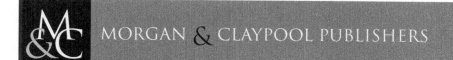

MORGAN & CLAYPOOL PUBLISHERS

ABSTRACT

Performing fieldwork in healthcare settings is significantly different from fieldwork in other domains and it presents unique challenges to researchers. Whilst results are reported in research papers, the details of how to actually perform these fieldwork studies are not.

This is the first of two volumes designed as a collective graduate guidebook for conducting fieldwork in healthcare. This volume brings together the experiences of established researchers who do fieldwork in clinical and non-clinical settings, focusing on how people interact with healthcare technology, in the form of case studies. These case studies are all personal, reflective accounts of challenges faced and lessons learned, which future researchers might also learn from.

We open with an account of studies in the Operating Room, focusing on the role of the researcher, and how participants engage and resist engaging with the research process. Subsequent case studies address themes in a variety of hospital settings, which highlight the variability that is experienced across study settings and the importance of context in shaping what is possible when conducting research in hospitals. Recognising and dealing with emotions, strategies for gaining access, and data gathering are themes that pervade the studies.

Later case studies introduce research involving collaborative design and intervention studies, which seek to have an immediate impact on practice. Mental health is a theme of two intervention studies as we move out of the hospital to engage with vulnerable participants suffering from long-term conditions and people in the home. This volume closes with an intervention study in the developing world that ends with some tips for conducting studies in healthcare. Such tips are synthesised through the thematic chapters presented in the companion volume.

KEYWORDS

fieldwork, healthcare, ethnography, medical devices, HCI, human-computer interaction, health, methodology, case studies

Contents

8   Deploying Healthcare Technology "in the wild:" Experiences from Deploying a Mobile Health Technology for Bipolar Disorder Treatment

Mads Frost and Steven Houben

Anja Thieme, Paula Johnson, Jayne Wallace, Patrick Olivier, and Thomas D. Meyer

Preface

Dominic Furniss, Aisling Ann O'Kane, Rebecca Randell, Svetlena Taneva, Helena Mentis, and Ann Blandford, (Editors)

INTRODUCTION

Conducting fieldwork for investigating human factors and technology use in healthcare is a challenging undertaking, and yet there is little in the way of community support and guidance for conducting these studies. Although results are published in research papers, there is little room to describe methodological challenges, solutions, study experience, advice, and guidance. The motivation for these two volumes on fieldwork for investigating human factors and computing systems in healthcare is to share experience and guidance within the broader community as well as with future researchers. The focus is on the experiences of the fieldwork researcher, without medical training, who may be studying technology design or work practices (e.g., to improve patient safety); it is not on that of clinicians and patients who bring complementary perspectives to the research.

This first volume, which presents 12 case studies, emphasises the sharing of challenges and strategies from experienced researchers. The second complementary volume presents six chapters of advice and guidance for researchers who are planning and conducting fieldwork to investigate the use of technology in healthcare. Both books are intended as a resource for those interested in teaching and learning how to conduct fieldwork in healthcare. They can inform new researchers' project plans and contingency plans in this complex and challenging domain. For more experienced researchers, this volume offers advice and support through familiar stories and experiences. For lecturers and supervisors, it offers a source of reference and debate.

BACKGROUND

The idea for these volumes first arose through reflecting on the challenges we experienced with planning and conducting fieldwork in healthcare on a project at UCL (University College London). With little guidance from any published literature we had to learn hard and fast on the job as we encountered different challenges and issues unique to the domain. One source of support was sharing stories with people involved in similar activities whom we met at conferences and the like: similar issues were recognised, advice was shared, and confidence was gained in knowing that we were not alone or wrongly conducting the work.

This pooling of knowledge turned into a more formal approach when a larger group of us came together to write a paper on the challenges of doing Human-Computer Interaction (HCI) fieldwork in healthcare "in the wild." The experience of sharing the challenges we faced and strategies we took to overcome those challenges was both rewarding and productive. Many of us had not had the opportunity to share these experiences in such a manner before. We benefited from this small community support and we all recognised the need to help ourselves and others learn from these experiences. There was a desire to expand this activity to the broader community and so we organised a workshop at the ACM Conference on Human Factors in Computing Systems (CHI), the aim of which was to produce a graduate guidebook for those undertaking fieldwork for the purpose of designing and/or evaluating healthcare technologies.

The editors of this volume got together and organised a workshop on April 27, 2013. A subset of the submissions were edited and are included in this volume of the book. The activities of the workshop itself provided an opportunity to generate a set of common issues, which became the structure for the second volume on guidance. Consequently, this whole project has involved many people from our international research community, and the diversity of their perspectives brings benefit to both volumes.

Even though these case studies draw from a HCI perspective we were strongly advised that these issues would have broader appeal to people in neighbouring disciplines, e.g., ergonomics, informatics, psychology, biomedical engineering, etc. Consequently, we preferred "human factors in computing systems" as a broader title to capture the focus of the material but maintain the breadth of issues we have covered for neighbouring disciplines. This also firmly keeps our roots in the workshop at CHI.

We take a broad view of fieldwork and healthcare. Fieldwork refers to those techniques that require the researcher to gather data "in the wild" which contrasts with surveys and laboratory studies. Fieldwork commonly involves some form of observation or interview in context. Our view of healthcare is also broad and includes clinical contexts like hospitals, non-clinical contexts like home healthcare, mental health, preventative medicine, and care.

OVERVIEW: A TOUR OF THE STYLE, STRUCTURE, AND CONTENT

Style

When planning this book we wanted to move away from a dry academic style of reporting to recreate something more like the conversations that we had with one another. We wanted to bring experiences to life through sharing stories, which could be enlightening, sad, or even amusing. Consequently, we have encouraged a personal and confessional style of reporting which helps place the reader in the situation of the author and closer to their experience. This goes beyond methodological concerns to include how the researchers felt about the situation they were in. In these case studies you will encounter a diversity of experiences, cultures and practices. Readers should be mindful of extracting absolute generalizable lessons from single accounts: just because one author found it hard to engage with clinicians does not mean you will; just because one author encountered a strong blame culture in healthcare does not mean you will; and if someone has not followed best practice it does not mean you should do the same. All of these experiences should be understood relative to their context, at that time, for that author, and for that project. Guidance is drawn together and offered in a companion volume.

Structure

This book is roughly divided into two parts. The first part presents relatively traditional observational studies in hospital settings, while the second part focuses on designing interventions and observational studies outside the hospital context. Chapters 1–3 present detailed examples of the issues that can be uncovered through fieldwork in hospital. Chapters 4–6 present considerations for the researcher in conducting fieldwork in healthcare around particular themes. Chapters 7–9 move on to addressing the challenges of designing interventions in hospital and for people with mental health issues. Chapters 10–11 cover practical and methodological issues in the home. Chapter 12 takes us further away from home by looking at significant health issues in the developing world through the review of an intervention study on a maternity ward in Nairobi, Kenya.

Content

Each chapter provides insights and communicates a deep understanding of the opportunities and challenges of doing fieldwork in healthcare.

In Chapter 1, Sellen et al. take us straight into the practicalities of setting up a detailed evaluation of new technology in healthcare. The technology was an Electronic Remote Blood Issue system, which issues units of blood remotely from the blood bank department. The authors detail their experiences of gathering data from three urban hospitals. Their account covers the challenge of evaluating technology that is used infrequently and sporadically, setting up video recording equipment, managing ethics, and access, and conflict with different groups and cultures.

Sarcevic grapples with trying to understand trauma resuscitation as a socio-technical system in Chapter 2. Here, we learn more about managing access and ethical issues. Through the narrative about this multi-site study, we find that hospitals have different expectations and scope of acceptable study methods, e.g., some allowed video data collection and others did not. What makes this chapter stand out is the extreme environment that the research is performed in and the emotional, practical, and intellectual challenges that come with that.

In Chapter 3, Furniss brings us into a less dynamic environment but one where death and critically ill patients are common: an oncology ward. Compared to the first two chapters, the starting point is exploratory and a big issue for the author is finding the right research focus. He questions whether the right focus is the one that leads towards a successful research paper or the one that engages with a significant practical issue for the ward. The author highlights the role of research champions who can unlock data, insights, and issues related to engaging with staff and patients on the ward.

Chapter 4 is the first of three chapters that draw out significant themes from all of the details of practice. Chagpar and colleagues identify different emotional situations that researchers can find themselves in: observing people in vulnerable situations, situations we perceive as dangerous, and isolated fragments of complex medical processes. Emotion is a theme that stretches throughout the book as healthcare so often deals with people that are vulnerable or at risk due to their health condition. The flip side is that this is what makes work in healthcare so important: it has the potential for significant impact on people's lives and wellbeing.

In Chapter 5, Randell draws our attention to the theme of finding balance. The case study focuses on experiences of doing a multi-site study of patient handovers in hospitals. We get a feel for the long days that fieldwork takes, the awkwardness of approaching patients and family members to provide informed consent at sensitive times, and the emotions involved in hearing about unfortunate news and witnessing sad events. Compounding these challenges were the intellectual and practical problems of finding where handovers happen and negotiating how to study these. Rightly, the author highlights that we need to find balance in our studies: between the ethics committees and the demands of the research, between the research and the researcher, and between time for data collection and time for analysis. It is easy to get swept up by all the challenges of doing this type of work, so we need to take our time to plan, find the right approach, and balance the competing demands of the project.

In Chapter 6, Hilligoss draws our attention to the theme of access. Complementing Chapter 5, this case study details experiences of studying patient handover and hospital admissions. In this study, we learn of the importance of networking in opening doors and gaining access. The author attempted to access different perspectives and different data but not all of these ventures were successful. As in the case study reported in Chapter 3, the author tried but eventually gave up on interviewing an entire clinician group. Practical considerations are described as well, such as what you should wear in the target environment and how you should present yourself. This chapter is a reminder to expect surprises and to be flexible in your work.

Chapter 7 by Groth and Frykholm is a great example of how healthcare professionals and HCI professionals can work together, in contrast to case studies that present the difficulties of such engagement. This study does the opposite: it demonstrates how one can achieve great collaboration with healthcare professionals and engages them in the design processes (e.g., design workshops, prototyping sessions, and evaluations). One of the success factors is to have a key figure of influence supporting the work. More broadly, this highlights the importance of the organisational context and history your project starts within, which can greatly affect the potential cooperation you do or do not get.

Frost and Houben (Chapter 8) present another case study covering design and intervention. It is the first of two studies concerned with mental healthcare, focusing on developing a smart phone app for people with bipolar disorder. This case study emphasises the practicalities you need to consider to make novel interventions work when you are evaluating them in healthcare. This includes setting up mobile phone contracts with patients, helping them with technological issues broader than the projects scope, setting up a helpline in case there are unforeseen issues, etc. The chapter ends with interesting reflections on the unintended effects of technology deployment: access to new data meant new responsibility and new concerns for the changing job role of the clinicians involved.

Chapter 9 by Thieme et al. is also a design study in a mental health context but differs in that it covers the creative processes and describes the extremely vulnerable people who take part in the study. The patients are women who are kept in a secure unit because of personality disorders. The key to working in this extreme environment is collaboration. As healthcare technology researchers and designers, we are outside our comfort zone in such environments and have to rely on clinicians to advise us, collaborate with us, and chaperone us so that we, and the people we work with, remain safe. This case study provides a fascinating account of how a creative project was managed in this extreme context.

Building on examples of studies outside of the hospital, Chapter 10 by Thomson et al. focuses on the challenges of interviewing older people in their homes. One of the main issues, which reminds us of the access issue in the preceding studies, is recruitment. For example, how do you identify and recruit appropriate members of a sub-population who are dispersed around the community? We are reminded of the practicalities of remaining safe when doing fieldwork away from fixed professional establishments and get tips on interviewing people in their homes about their health issues.

In Chapter 11, Rajkomar et al. complement the methodological advice of the previous chapter. Focusing on investigating the design and use of home haemodialysis technology, the authors report on their attempts to use a number of user research techniques such as video and paper diaries that are not effective. Adapting to the context, they eventually settled on situated critical incident interviews as an appropriate and fruitful way to gather data, which balances the needs of the research, the researcher and the patient. Further examples of adaptability are shown through the account of having to abandon some of the research pursuits due to organisational changes beyond the control of the authors. Critically, the authors bring to our attention that patients rely on these medical devices to maintain independent living and appearing competent in using them provides them such sense of independence. This has knock-on implications when trying to elicit usability problems.

Finally, Chapter 12 by Underwood moves us toward considering major world-wide health issues. The case study details the introduction of a new technology to a maternity ward in Nairobi, Kenya. The new technology is designed to facilitate the use of the World Health Organisation's guidance to help detect serious maternal and foetal complications during labour. The author has very practical tips that apply as much to healthcare contexts that are closer to home as they do to this context: budgeting for extra time, adding value to the workplace you are in, putting your pride aside when taking feedback, and setting some personal goals that are different from your research goals.

Overall, this volume presents personal experiences and lessons learned with a case study approach. The companion volume *Fieldwork in Healthcare: Guidance for Studies in Human Factors and Computer Systems* is a guidebook that distils best practices and principles for conducting fieldwork in healthcare—from project planning and getting access to a clinical environment, to research dissemination and stakeholder management. These are complementary volumes.

Acknowledgements

This volume has been a pleasure to guide and produce. It started as a seed of an idea and has grown into a lasting contribution. Along the way we have shared and learnt a lot, and at last some of this is in print for others to engage with, debate, and learn from too. We hope researchers will be informed and inspired by some of these case studies, that more experienced researchers will be able to find support and advice, and that teachers will be able to use this material for instruction and debate.

Many people from across geographical boundaries contributed to these two volumes. We would like to thank all who contributed, both directly through case studies and indirectly through support in making this project happen. We would particularly like to thank the committee who supported our workshop proposal and helped us review its submissions. We would like to thank all of our workshop participants for making the event a success. We would also like to thank Ron Baecker and Diane Cerra, on the publishing side, for their support and advice.

WORKSHOP COMMITTEE

Gregory Abowd, Jonathan Back, Ken Catchpole, Gavin Doherty, Geraldine Fitzpatrick, Ioanna (Jo) Iacovides, Josette Jones, Tom Owen, Madhu Reddy, Mark Rouncefield, Penelope Sanderson, Chris Vincent, Robert Wears, and Stephanie Wilson.

WORKSHOP PARTICIPANTS

Anjum Chagpar, Deborah Chan, Yunan Chen, Andy Dearden, Mads Frost, Kristina Groth, Brian Hilligoss, Cecily Morrison, Atish Rajkomar, Raj Ratwani, Aleksandra Sarcevic, Katherine Sellen, Anja Thieme, Ross Thomson, Heather Underwood, and Xiaomu Zhou.

FUNDING

The first, second, and last editor were funded by the CHI+MED project, supported by the UK Engineering and Physical Sciences Research Council [EPSRC grant reference EP/G059063/1].

CHAPTER 1

Confessions from the Operating Suite: Negotiating Capture, Resistance, Errors, and Identity

Katherine Sellen, Mark Chignell, Jeannie Callum, Jacob Pendergrast, and Alison Halliday

Healthcare settings can pose particular challenges when conducting research on adoption and adaptation to new technologies, especially when medical errors are a subject of the research, or the research necessitates capturing user behaviours and interactions. This chapter describes a multi-site evaluation of an Electronic Remote Blood Issue system, conducted in the operating suites and blood banks of three urban hospitals. Particular issues that the chapter explores include:

- Capturing data related to events that happen infrequently;

- Getting ethical approval for video capture and the practical issues in setting that up; and

- Managing research participants' acts of resistance.

1.1   RESEARCH FOCUS

Healthcare settings present a particularly challenging research domain for Human-Computer Interaction (HCI). There is increasing evidence from evaluation studies of Health Information Technologies (HIT) that there are significant barriers to successful implementation that constitutes a gaping socio-technical gap. This gap often results in adaptation and adoption/abandonment that may be described as resistance to change and resistance to technology (Bardram, 1997; Jasperset al., 2008; Zheng, et al., 2005). The study described in this chapter applied an HCI approach to understanding adaptation and adoption/abandonment processes for a blood unit issue system designed to provide blood units for transfusion in operating suites.

The aim of this study was to investigate the potential relationship between use and experience of an HIT system and adaptation and adoption/abandonment processes. This included the experience of errors at the interface and medically relevant errors.

The blood issue system was chosen because of its relative simplicity compared to more complex HIT systems such as provider order entry or medical record systems. As such, it was expected that it could provide an opportunity for analysing a relatively small number of error types and behaviours, with which to investigate adaptation and adoption/abandonment processes. This was achieved through studying changing work practices, task sharing/shifting between roles, and human error with the introduction of a blood issue system at three urban hospitals over three years. The work practices and tasks tracked included the decision to transfuse, timing of blood retrieval, blood labeling, double checking, storage practices, the retrieval of units and number of units tranfused, wastage of blood, error recovery behaviours, and learning behaviours, among others. The implementation of the blood issue system at three different hospitals in short sucession proved very convenient for our research: more natural comparisons could be made that would have been difficult to fund and organise purely as a research initiative.

1.2   STUDY DESIGN

The study utilised a mixed methods approach informed by socio-technical perspectives on HIT implementation and evaluation (Berg et al., 2003). Errors (both medically relevant and recoverable errors at the interface), changing work practices, and adaptation/adoption/abandonment behavior were analysed and interpreted within the socio-technical context. The study design can be summarised as follows.

- **Site:** The operating suites and blood banks of three urban hospitals.

- **Technology:** Electronic Remote Blood Issue (ERBI) system for the remote issuing of blood units for transfusion to patients during surgery. The system consists of a database linked to the blood bank for tracking patient blood type and blood unit status, a kiosk, scanner, and label printer in the operating suite. This is connected to a fridge that it controls, which contains unmatched blood units located away from the blood bank close to the operating room (see Figure 1.1). This sytem replaced a manual system of blood order and delivery provided through the blood banks at the respective hospitals.

- **Participants:** All staff of the blood bank and operating teams were potential participants in the study, including laboratory staff, blood bank technicians, blood bank managers, physicians, anaesthesiologists, respiratory therapists, nurses, porters, and patient support staff.

- **Data collection:** Fieldwork was conducted over three years between 2008–2011, and included collection of qualitative and quantitative user survey data, formal and informal interviews with managers and staff, six weeks of observation at each site with 24 h video capture and in-person observation, and analysis of software log data. Incident reports, implementation-planning documents, and user feedback and troubleshooting log books were also accessed.

1.3   STUDY EXPERIENCE

Carrying out the study was a rich learning experience for the researchers and clinicians involved and several key experiences are described in this chapter from the perspective of the main researcher. These experiences illustrate a tension between the needs of a research study, the risks associated with something new, and the reality of change for clinicians engaged in the safety critical act of blood transfusion.

1.3.1   CAPTURING PATTERNS OF ACTIVITY

After initial meetings with the physician leaders at the three hospitals involved in the technology implementation, I spent a few weeks meeting with staff and looking around the spaces where the technology implementation would occur. I began to realise that studying the adoption of this technology was going to be quite a challenge. The activities that I would be studying did not follow a predictable pattern of working hours but could occur at any time of day or night; they could be once every 45 min or once every 7 days, and might last anywhere between 55 s and 45 min. Added to this was the realisation that each hospital had a slightly different case mix and therefore a slightly different pattern of activities. These activities ranged from the routine of knee and gall bladder surgery, the unpredictability of transplant surgery, to the diversity of trauma cases. Medical errors of interest to the study might occur once every six to nine months. I grasped that traditional ethnographic or observational techniques, either using human observers or handheld video recording, would be impractical.

Thankfully, the implementations at the three hospitals would not occur simultaneously but in sequence. This study needed to be designed so that it did not necessitate the continuous presence of an observer and worked within a number of other constraints, including:

- Unpredictable start times;

- Round the clock activity;

- Wide ranging activity durations and frequencies;

- Active or moving tasks;

- Frequent changes in personnel;

- Presence of patients and their significant others;

- Security concerns; and

- Infection control restrictions.

I realised that a combination of different data types including log files and video might be useful if we could find the right type of equipment. This could be combined with questionnaires, interviews, and in-person observations, to provide context and qualitative insight to the patterns uncovered in the log files and video.

1.3.2   VIDEO CAPTURE

I started with an Internet search for video capture and discovered some freeware developed as a hacked surveillance system using a cheap webcam for security concerned condo owners. I tried it out in the blood bank of the first site. Positioning the camera and laptop was a problem. It drew a lot of attention from staff. I inadvertently dislodged a ceiling tile that prompted a visit and warning from Infection Control. It soon became obvious that installing a webcam and leaving my laptop in the semi-public space of the operating suite was not an option. While looking for possible video equipment I chanced upon some surveillance systems for retail stores. The surveillance system used motion sensing and secured encrypted hard drives for storage. These systems were also set up for multiple cameras with different viewing angles (see Figure 1.1). This became a key piece of the study and is described in full elsewhere (Sellen et al., 2010). Working with a small budget, using technology designed for a comepletely different purpose was an unexpected success, and a lesson I put to use for future research.

1.3.3   APPROVAL FOR CAPTURE

Researchers who report on their research experiences in medical settings often document challenges posed by the medico-legal environment of hospitals. Staff may be resistant to having events captured in detail in case a medical error occurs, the legal department may be unwilling for errors and near misses to be recorded, and capturing identifiable data must be avoided (Gelbart et al., 2009). The issues of how to inform participants, obtain consent, and manage communication with participants can become a barrier to research (Mackenzie et al., 2007). In order to develop an ethical research protocol I conducted a review of published accounts of the use of video in healthcare settings. I then summarised this work into a special section for the Research Ethics Boards (REB). The REB invited me to a face-to-face meeting to discuss the study and this gave me an opportunity to show the equipment and talk through the procedures I was proposing. The REB process was lengthy and extensive, including three separate hospital REB reviews and my own home University REB review. I discussed using video with my research partners at the different hospitals. They then talked to their staff members and provided me with feedback about staff concerns. The front line staff managers in the blood banks were key partners in facilitating the use of video. They helped to ensure front line staff were comfortable and ensured staff would be unsurprised when cameras were installed and I started to take notes on their activities. Front line staff managers were also essential for when cameras were installed in the operating suites. I talked to front line staff weeks and then days in advance of cameras being installed, talked over the protocol several times and made myself available in confidence for questions. The response to the use of video was generally positive with some exceptions. I did discover that some nursing staff were disconnecting the video recording devices from their power sources, so I had to keep coming back to the operating suites to check the equipment, and after several weeks this stopped happening. It is possible that this was an act of resistance to the research on the part of the operating suite nurses. It is also possible that the way in which consent works for video capture in team settings still needs refining.

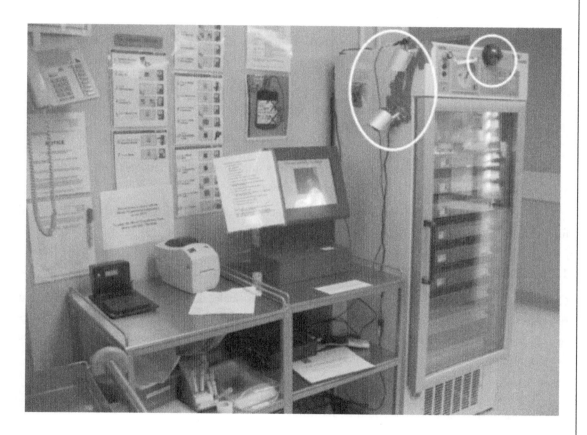

Figure 1.1: Example of video set-up in the operating suite showing two light gray cameras attached to the side of the fridge and one black fisheye camera above the fridge door.

1.3.4   STRATEGIES FOR RESEARCH ETHICS BOARDS (REB)

For developing an ethically workable video capture protocol, one that is acceptable to participants as well as the needs of the research, there are several strategies that the experience of this study would suggest.

- **Participation:** Identify and involve key stakeholders in the research design and in the implementation of the study.

- **Evidence:** Find precedents from published approved studies conducted either in the same institution or elsewhere.

- **Role-play:** Before you finalise the protocol, test out the proposed protocol using role-play or scenarios. This will help to uncover unexpected risks and practical considerations.

- **Demonstration:** Be prepared to show the REB the equipment you are proposing and demonstrate the protocols you will use.

- **Timelines:** Build in extra time for unusual protocols or new research designs.

- **Communication:** Make sure your participants and those who manage them are fully aware of the protocol before and during the research.

Advice and guidelines on research governance, ethics, and data gathering are developed further in Volume 2.

1.3.5   RESISTANCE TO RESEARCH

One of the challenges encountered in studying HCI in healthcare settings is the potential that resistance to technology, or resistance to change in general, will transform into resistance to research. I encountered many forms of resistance when carrying out the research activities in the field, including:

- Verbal intimidation;

- Suggesting activities that could be harmful;

- Spoiling of data collection sheets;

- Physical tampering with equipment; and

- Boycotting research.

I will elaborate on two of these. The nursing staff at one of the three sites made a group decision not to take part in the questionnaire and interview sections of the study. At a staff-wide meeting, where I introduced myself and presented the study, I was questioned by several senior nurses in front of a crowded room. They questioned the need for basic demographic data and accused me of ageism and racism (the questionnaire asked for age range and participant's first language). At first I interpreted this resistance to the study as a reflection of the lack of engagement of nursing staff in the development of the research agenda and I started to wonder how I might include nursing leaders in the development of the research. However, I suspected a decision not to participate had been made by the notional leaders of the group rather than senior managers. I decided to sit through the rest of the nursing meeting to see if this was the general style of things or whether this style had been reserved for me. I noticed that the same few senior nurses also dominated other presentations by fellow nurses. The majority of the nurses said nothing. My suspicions were confirmed when the official nurse leader divulged, in a private meeting, that she had no influence on perceptions of the research study by her staff. Separately, a nurse who had attended the meeting approached me. She explained that she had just joined the team from another hospital and understood what I was trying to do, that the research was needed, and that any help they could get to reduce errors should be embraced but that *the nurses here don't understand, they are years behind.* The group-wide response was clear direct resistance. I still wonder if a more participatory approach to research design could have helped but it is also possible that the culture of this particular nursing group was hostile to change in general.

Indirect resistance was more difficult to navigate. At one site, I was invited by a senior nurse to come with her into an operating room while an operation was in progress. She suggested that I distribute questionnaires directly inside the operating room even though this was clearly against the ethics protocol and would have been disruptive to the progress of the surgery, potentially threatening the patient's safety. This could have led to the suspension of the study at the hospital. I declined her invitation. I began to seriously doubt the design of the study and my ability as a researcher until I was informed several months later, *"We like the new system now, we* [the nursing staff] *were quite upset when it went off line the other day. If you do the questionnaires now I am sure people will fill them in. I can also arrange some interviews for you."*

I also learnt that the resistance was not only directed at the research activities but also towards the IT department and the blood bank. I observed that the system I was studying was described as *"blood bank technology."* This showed divisions between clinical specialties, which played a major role in resistance to the research. For example, at one point a disagreement between nursing and haematology over a JPEG image of a blood unit on the kiosk interface was elevated to a high-level committee at the hospital drawing negative attention to the blood bank and the technology initiative as a whole—our research was tied into, and affected by, these political divisions and disagreements.

1.3.6   RESEARCHING MEDICAL ERROR

Researching medical error can be a difficult undertaking. I knew from my previous research using video that medical error was a sensitive topic for research (Gelbart et al., 2009). However, I was surprised at the depth of reaction to errors and near misses when they did occur. One day, on entering the break room, I approached some nursing staff at a lunch table. They began to joke "*here comes the FBI.*" A nurse sitting alone nearby turned her face to the window when I approached. No one would talk to me. I heard someone mutter a question to another, "*Are we talking about it?*" "*No.*" came the response. I later learnt from one of the blood bank staff that a nurse had been involved in a serious near miss with the technology that I was studying that same week and the nurse involved had gone on medical leave from stress. Clearly, none of the front line staff involved were willing to talk about the incident. On a separate occasion while I was visiting the blood bank at another site, my key research partner told me what happened: "*…they have nurses crying in the corridors too afraid to use the technology in case they make a mistake and too afraid to go back into the room because they will be shouted at.*" I was not expecting there to be a hostile culture in the hospitals where the study was conducted but I have since discovered that this is commonplace (Hutchinson et al., 2006).

A sense of shame and fear of consequences seemed to characterise the conversations about errors that I was able to achieve during the main part of the study. I went to talk to the anaesthesiologists at one site about their experience of the new technology. One anaesthesiologist remarked, "*I don't know why the blood bank gets so anxious about us taking units out. What's the big deal?*" I explained that the units were not cross-matched until the labels had been printed and the units scanned. A look of horror crept over his face as he realised that he had removed blood for transfusion that had not been cross-matched and he looked at the table. He did not participate in the rest of the session. I realised I had inadvertently exposed his error in front of his colleagues, but I also felt an obligation to explain the potential for serious error to him and his colleagues when he posed his question. I also found myself shielding nursing staff from scrutiny when video footage from the study showed deviations from procedures that could have led to patient misidentification. I adopted a strategy of only discussing aggregate data, describing types of errors rather than specific errors.

I realised that fixing the culture of blame, shame, and punishment in the settings I found myself in was out of scope for my research, but that my research activities had the potential to inform safety initiatives if handled in a sensitive way. After several years of working on the study, no one had been blamed, shamed, or punished as a result of my involvement and so I was able to work more freely on the topic of error. For example, I was given access to error reports and I was able to provide specific recommendations for design modifications that would enhance safety.

1.3.7   IDENTITY

Many different people move around the research setting, some are directly involved in the research and others are not. In different settings in the hospitals where I have worked my identity is interpreted in different ways and that identity has meaning in terms of status, resources conferred, and data provisioned. When in the operating suite I am usually mistaken for a junior nurse, never a physician or a surgeon. My activities were questioned, my behaviour and equipment scrutinised. In the blood bank I am usually mistaken for a medical resident. The lab technicians participate somewhat willingly in the research, but some resent my involvement. I suspect that the perception of my level in the hierarchy, my gender, age, and what I wear plays a part in this. In the operating suite I am dressed as a nurse but the items I wear do not bear the hallmarks of years of professional practice. In the blood bank I can wear my regular research clothes. I am not encouraged to wear a lab coat and so I cannot be mistaken for a blood bank technician. I have also become sensitive to the role of research in medical settings generally. It would be unusual for a junior nurse or a blood bank staff member to engage in research. This is the privilege of senior physician researchers and medical residents or fellows. Perceived as a junior nurse, I would have no claim to the researcher role. This may, in part, explain resistance to the research, however, my experience of resistance differed quite markedly between hospitals, despite making more or less the same choices in terms of dress. The majority of the resistance was experienced at the same site where bullying and shaming were most obvious. Themes of identity and reflexivity are discussed further in Volume 2: Chapter 2.

1.4   IMPLICATIONS FOR RESEARCHERS

From a theoretical perspective socio-technical theory is likely to be relevant in study design and analysis of any *in situ* HCI research in healthcare. With a socio-technical approach, mixed methods should be considered, and ethnographic techniques, such as researcher diaries, may aid in capturing relevant socio-technical context. Participatory engagement with each clinical specialty in study design may reduce resistance and maximize the likelihood of study success. In order to achieve study success with all of these elements in place, the timeline of the study development must be considered from the outset. REB approval and building rapport can take longer in healthcare settings and finding the right equipment can require some creative solutions. In addition, choice of clothing and accessories carries specific meaning in healthcare environments, a reality that researchers should be sensitive to when choosing to adopt the dress of their participants. Encountering cultures of bullying and shaming, especially around error, is an unfortunate reality for many clinical settings, and a reality that HCI researchers should be aware of when they plan research. Studies with longer timeframes will enable rapport building and trust to develop, which can mitigate some of these obstacles and positively impact data gathering.

1.5   CONCLUSION

Just as technology is experienced *in situ*, so is research. Plans need to be made and negotiated, which include capturing data, resistance to the research, managing error, and identity. In some sense the research is tied to the context within which it is being performed. The difference in response to the research between the three hospitals reflected the culture and political climate of each setting. This in turn was reflected in the adoption experience of the technology under study. This has practical and theoretical implications for human computer interaction, and highlights the need to reconsider the idea of resistance in experiences of adaptation, adoption, and abandonment of new technology, as well as resistance to research.

ACKNOWLEDGEMENT

This work was funded by a MITACS grant. We thank the staff at each of the three hospitals for their support and involvement in this study.

CHAPTER 2

Understanding Trauma Resuscitation: Experiences from the Field and Lessons Learned

Aleksandra Sarcevic

This chapter describes the experiences and lessons learned from fieldwork in the domain of trauma resuscitation conducted over seven years at several U.S. trauma centres. Particular issues that the chapter explores include:

- The process of getting access to research sites;

- Applying the language of medical ethics committees to the design of qualitative research protocols; and

- Undertaking observations in crowded, high-pressure environments.

2.1 RESEARCH FOCUS

Over the past seven years, our multidisciplinary research group has studied the work of medical teams during trauma resuscitation—a high-risk, fast-paced, and information-laden process of treating severely injured patients in a dedicated facility in the emergency department (Figure 2.1). The resuscitation process is one of the most demanding in healthcare, requiring the team of 7–15 medical professionals to focus on patient care for a short time period, while adapting to complex and changing circumstances driven by patient status (Barach & Weinger, 2007).

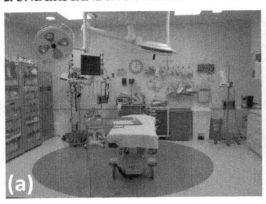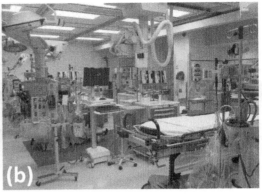

Figure 2.1: Example trauma bays at our research sites (a, b).

Our long-term research goal has been the design and development of a context-aware system that monitors the work of trauma teams, and alerts them to errors and process deviations associated with adverse outcomes. Conceptualizing such a system required a careful study of the work processes (e.g., team communications and interactions, decision making, leadership, errors) using several approaches, including fieldwork. To date, we have conducted studies at, and collaborated with, three urban, highest-level U.S. trauma centres, two of which are paediatric: Children's National Medical Centre (CNMC), Washington, DC; The Children's Hospital of Philadelphia (CHOP), Philadelphia, PA; and Robert Wood Johnson University Hospital (RWJ), New Brunswick, NJ. The studies involved fieldwork (i.e., participant observation, interviews, shadowing); video review of real and simulated resuscitation events; and design, development, and evaluation of technology prototypes using participatory design. As a member of our research group who has been responsible for designing and conducting field studies, in this case study I discuss several themes and challenges that we encountered in our work, including access to research sites, project management, study design and ethics, fieldwork experiences, and collaboration with clinicians.

2.2   ACCESS AND PROJECT MANAGEMENT

Access to research sites and project management are tightly coupled because they both depend on the working relationship with medical collaborators (see Volume 2: Chapter 3 for more information). An ideal case would involve medical collaborators who could dedicate a substantial amount of their time to managing research at the site, assisting with grant applications, co-authoring manuscripts, and participating in the research. Finding such collaborators, however, is difficult. For example, trauma resuscitation as a discipline lies within the realms of emergency medicine and general surgery. Because trauma patients require many resources, some trauma centres have designated trauma teams whose sole responsibility is taking care of trauma patients. Yet many hospitals do not have such capabilities and members of the trauma team have other duties throughout the day (e.g., surgeries, emergency care, critical care, etc.), which makes their involvement in research less likely.

Although our research sites were not dedicated trauma centres, they were located in urban, teaching hospitals with established research infrastructures and mechanisms that allow medical personnel to conduct research. We were fortunate to find dedicated collaborators at most of our sites. Two factors contributed to this success. First, we conceptualised our research program to have an impact not only within the HCI and engineering fields, but also on improving patient care, allowing our medical collaborators to become vital stakeholders. They saw an opportunity to develop their own research agendas within the projects' scopes; they were able to extend their roles from collaborators to project co-investigators and even principal investigators, leading aspects of the research that were patient-centred rather than technology- or design-centred. This arrangement allowed our medical collaborators to be independent yet accountable, as well as to have budgets for managing research at the sites (e.g., paying research coordinators to assist with participant recruitment and ethical approvals, buying equipment, covering participants' expenses, etc.). Second, most of our collaborators are physician-researchers or division chiefs with a significant percentage of their time research-protected (e.g., 75% research time and 25% clinical time). Depending on the hospital, protected research time may also mean physicians having responsibility for securing additional funding to cover for their research time. This factor has played a crucial role in our research because it further motivated medical experts to work with us.

Having established such working relationships with our collaborators made it easier to obtain access to research sites, healthcare personnel, and events of interest. For each site, I received a hospital badge and a pager (Figure 2.2). Because the pager is used to notify trauma teams of an incoming patient, I found it especially useful during observational periods; if in close proximity, I was able to arrive to the trauma bay in time to observe real events. Most helpful, however, was the arrangement with one of the hospitals where I spent six months working as a volunteer. I had a dedicated desk in the office adjacent to the emergency department, shared with personnel involved in research and administrative aspects of trauma resuscitation. I often refer to this arrangement as my "research residency" since it allowed me to (a) spend as much time as I needed in the hospital; (b) understand not only the domain of interest but also the hospital life in general; (c) meet with medical experts and personnel from different departments and disciplines; and (d) collect rich data.

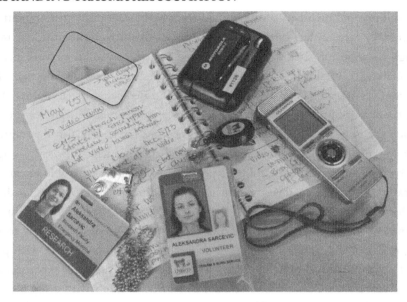

Figure 2.2. Tools of the trade: Notebook, audio recorder, hospital badges, pager, and photo camera (used to capture this photograph).

2.3   STUDY DESIGNS AND ETHICAL ISSUES

Study designs varied depending on the focus of a study, which ranged from understanding teamwork, decision making, leadership, communication, and process deviations and errors. Most studies involved real-time observations of actual and simulated resuscitations, interviews with trauma team members, and shadowing. Some studies also involved analysis of team interactions using video review of both simulated and actual resuscitations. We also conducted participatory design workshops to solicit expert opinion about technology designs (see Volume 2: Chapter 4 for more information on data gathering techniques). Rather than having one ethical approval covering the entire research program, we obtained ethical approval for each study. Although this approach was time consuming, it provided some flexibility in conducting research. For example, research protocols involving observation and interviews required a less rigorous, exempt review, which is typically performed within a week or two. Protocols involving video recording of real resuscitations, on the other hand, required the most rigorous, full ethical review. By dividing research into several protocols, we were able to start with some portions of the research while still waiting for the approvals for more complex parts.

Ethical approvals were needed from both the hospitals and our own academic institutions. We first obtained approvals from the hospitals and then applied for university approvals. Most recently, however, we switched to obtaining *IRB (Institutional Review Board) Authorization Agree-*

ments[1] rather than applying for separate university approvals. These agreements allow the hospital to act as the approval of record for another institution. The agreements also obviate the need for a committee review at another institution and so help speed up the process.

Even so, obtaining ethical approvals at the hospitals was not simple. Each hospital had a different set of requirements and protocols that needed to be followed. Depending on the study, it took between a few weeks to several months to obtain approvals. Ethics committees at hospitals are used to reviewing research protocols involving rigorous experimental designs and clinical trials, making our exploratory and social science-based protocols quite challenging to prepare. For example, it was difficult and sometimes inappropriate to try to calculate sample size or power, or specify primary and secondary endpoints for exploratory, observational studies. Similarly, it was difficult to anticipate the number of participatory workshops and simulations needed to reach usable technology designs. Over time and through the help of our medical collaborators, we learned how to adopt the language of the medical ethics committee and apply it to our protocols. Although written in medical research jargon, these protocols did not impact our actual study designs; adapting our language to that of ethics committees meant medical ethics committees could understand them better. For example, the protocol to assess the feasibility of a technology prototype in a simulation setting included the following paragraph about sample size and power:

> *"This is a pilot study. We will not have enough simulation sessions to power our primary endpoint to find the difference in the percent of team situation awareness with each intervention, as well as to power our secondary endpoints to find a difference in time to critical interventions and changes in workload. We will use this data to power our next study phase, which will likely require participation from multiple sites. We decided to plan for six simulation scenarios for this pilot study, based on time and participants available at this single site. However, we may determine the need to run more or less simulations based on our experience with initial simulation scenarios."*

The most challenging protocols we filed to date were the ones in which we requested video recording of actual resuscitations and a waiver of informed consent. One hospital approved our video recording protocol but denied the waiver of consent, requiring that we erase all video records within 96 h. To conduct research at this site, we collected consent forms from over 250 medical providers who typically participate in trauma resuscitations prior to the study; video review involved detailed transcriptions to preserve as much data as possible while meeting the 96-h limit. We had better luck at another hospital where video recording of actual resuscitations was already incorporated as part of the performance improvement process, so we piggybacked onto this practice. We were also able to obtain the waiver of informed consent by better explaining how our research met the standards for a Waiver, as defined by the Health and Human Services Secretary's Advisory

---

[1] IRB stands for Institutional Review Board in the U.S., and is an equivalent to Research Ethics Committees in other countries.

Committee on Human Research Protections (2008). In particular, following the guidelines defined by this Advisory Committee, we listed the following reasons for the waiver.

1. The research involves no more than minimal risk.

"Trauma team members will not be identified in transcriptions of trauma resuscitations. In addition, information that would permit direct or indirect identification of trauma team members will not be included. Patients will similarly not be identified. Protected health information (PHI), such as medical record number will be used only to link records to recordings and transcriptions of trauma resuscitations. After data linkages have been used, PHI will be removed from the data before analyses. Data linkages will be maintained on a password-protected computer and will be destroyed at the conclusion of the study."

2. The waiver will not adversely affect the rights and welfare of the participants.

"Video recordings and data transcribed from these recordings, as well as patient data, are now being collected and used for performance improvement purposes. As stated above, PHI will only be used for linking records and will be removed before analysis for research purposes."

3. The research could not practicably be carried out without the waiver.

"The individuals participating in trauma resuscitation are drawn from a large pool of potential individuals. The team includes providers from both inside and outside the hospital. In addition, the composition of the pool from which team members are drawn is dynamic, with new members being added or removed based on their assigned role rather than by their name. It is impractical to obtain consent from this large group of providers in advance. Even if possible to obtain consent in advance, requiring consent would decrease rather than increase the protection of privacy of participants. In our protocol, we will identify trauma team members only by their role, not their name. If consent were required, researchers would need to record the names of the team members to verify that those individuals had consented to participate in the study. Requiring consent would also threaten the scientific validity of the study by causing self-selection bias. The most likely practitioners to decline to participate would be those who are less confident about their role and responsibilities during the resuscitation. It is essential that resuscitations and teams of all types be included in our analysis."

2.4   EXPERIENCES FROM THE FIELD

Conducting fieldwork in a hospital's trauma unit is insightful but it also poses many challenges. Trauma resuscitations are relatively infrequent and random. On average, each of the sites treats about 500 trauma patients per year, with some days seeing more than one patient and some days passing without a single patient. Resuscitations are also more common during evening and night shifts, given the nature of traumatic injuries (e.g., gunshot or stabbing wounds, injuries caused by motor vehicle accidents or burns). Real observations were thus both physically and emotionally challenging. I was able to observe most events occurring during the day, while I was in the hospital. I also observed events occurring during a dozen or so nights I put on my schedule. Even so, it was difficult to balance the number of events observed during the day vs. night, resulting in a much larger, and somewhat skewed number of daily events available for analysis.

Another challenge were observations themselves. Trauma rooms are generally small and packed to capacity with medical equipment. The rooms are also crowded and noisy; on average, there were about 7–15 people per event, but this number increased as the severity of the patient injury increased—sometimes there were 20–30 people in one event, and exceptionally once there were 47 people. At first, it felt uncomfortable being there. I felt like I was obstructing someone's view or was in the clinicians' way. I would position myself in the corner, trying to occupy as little space as possible, but this positioning often compromised my ability to see things clearly. During observations, I would wear my badge and white coat to blend with the environment. But I would also carry my notebook to jot down notes, which made me stand out. At times, I even offered help—fetch a piece of equipment or make a phone call—to make myself useful. The emotional impact was hard, especially in the beginning, and while observing children. I was forcing myself to control emotions during observations, but pictures of injured patients came back in the evenings, when I was home, alone with my field notes and thoughts. Over time, I learned to view each patient as just another object of work, the strategy applied by many healthcare professionals. I was also sharing my experiences with trauma personnel in the office to better cope with these difficulties.

Like live observations, conducting interviews with trauma team members posed some challenges. Scheduling times for interviews was easier at the site where I did my research residency; I knew most of the care providers and was able to adjust to their busy schedules. Still, interviews varied in length and were often interrupted by pager notifications and calls for duty. Interviewing at the sites where I would visit for a few days a week to conduct observations was more challenging. To maximise my time during those visits, I would usually wait for the actual events in the emergency department near the nurses' station and interview trauma team members during idle times. These conversations, however, were also short with many interruptions.

In addition to observations and interviews, I also shadowed surgical residents during morning and afternoon rounds, and attended weekly surgical and emergency medicine conferences, performance improvement sessions, and mortality and morbidity meetings. Having access to these events was essential; discussions and reports shared during these meetings helped me to not only better understand the domain, but also to meet different people involved in general trauma care. Even with this level of access, getting to know every single care provider and establish rapport proved to be challenging for one simple reason: our sites are teaching hospitals with high staff turnover, especially residents. The high turnover also meant re-introducing myself each time a new group of residents or fellows arrived (every three to six months). Although our medical collaborators made every effort to introduce me to trauma team members, it was almost impossible to keep pace with the frequently changing social fabric at each site.

2.5   CONCLUSION

I will conclude with a short story and a lesson showing that regardless of the efforts we put into planning our field studies, there are always unanticipated contingencies that may interfere with our plans.

 At the end of my six-month residency at one of the sites, I gave a presentation at the monthly trauma meeting. I was both excited and intimidated by this opportunity because it allowed me to share the results of my work with an audience composed of general surgeons, emergency medicine physicians, fellows, and residents; at the time, it was the most critical audience I had ever presented to. I started the presentation by describing my educational and research background, the methods I had been using, and the insights I gained through fieldwork. After the presentation, one of the surgical fellows approached me and said: "*I wish you gave this presentation when you came here six months ago. I would have known you better and the reasons why you are here.*" This comment was an eye opener. Have I completed all this work with people barely knowing why I did it? Has this impacted the results I obtained? I was introducing myself and explaining the goals of my research many times throughout the fieldwork, sometimes even to the same people. Still, I realised it would have helped doing such presentations more often, perhaps each time a new cohort of residents arrived, or once a month, or after each round of preliminary results. It is my advice then to go back to the already busy clinicians regularly, not only for expert input or feedback on the results, but also to allow them to get to know us better.

ACKNOWLEDGEMENT

I would like to thank our medical collaborators at the research sites. Thanks also to the members of our research group (http://www.tru-it.rutgers.edu/). Our research has been supported by several NSF and NIH grants, including IIS-0915871, IIS-0915899, IIS-0915812, IIS-0803732, and R21LM011320-01A1.

CHAPTER 3

HCI Observations on an Oncology Ward: A Fieldworker's Experience

Dominic Furniss

This chapter presents reflections on the experience of doing a study on the design and use of medical devices on an Oncology Ward. It reports on a short study, carried out over 10 days and 4 nights, conducting observations and contextual interviews. The particular issues drawn out in this chapter are:

- Finding the research focus—whether to focus on the data we have access to or on the more interesting but infrequent events where we have little data;

- The role of "research champions" who can unlock fruitful data; and

- The reality and challenges of interacting with patients when shadowing staff.

3.1 RESEARCH FOCUS

I started to engage with the Oncology Ward after completing an observational study of an Oncology Day Care Unit (an outpatient unit), and before similar planned studies in a Haematology Ward and Intensive Therapy Unit (ITU). In all of these settings, the research focus was on the design and use of medical devices in context. The intention was to pay special attention to infusion pump use (a device used to pump fluids into patients), but the use of other interactive programmable medical devices was not excluded from the research. Part of my rationale was to investigate whether and how the design requirements of infusion pumps differed across contexts in hospitals but also more generally I wanted to find usability problems with medical devices, e.g., where nurses had difficulty with data entry and where interfaces could be designed to be more intuitive.

3.2 STUDY DESIGN

The study's design was an extension of the research I did in the Oncology outpatient unit, i.e., observations and interviews in context. I needed approval from the National Health Service (NHS) Research Ethics Committee (REC) for that original study, which took about four months to prepare (including a maze of advice and extensive forms; various meetings with clinical, management, and administrative staff; and signatures from multiple medical directors) and five months for it to be reviewed and approved. I submitted an amendment to extend the original approval to include the Oncology Ward, Haematology Ward, and ITU, which took just one month to be approved. Given these timeframes, requesting amendments for subsequent similar studies seems more efficient than submitting a new study proposal from scratch (see Volume 2: Chapter 2 for advice on ethics and governance).

As before, I would explain the study to staff at the beginning of every shift and get their consent through written forms. Any observations would be voluntary and I would work-shadow the nurses at appropriate times to see how medical devices were used. All staff and patients would remain anonymous in any written reports. The research protocol that was approved meant that the only time that anonymity would be compromised was if I felt that there was a patient safety concern and I needed to alert other members of staff to the situation.

I had access to hospital counsellors if I needed it, e.g., if I was disturbed by anything whilst I conducted my studies. This precaution was taken upon the recommendation of an experienced healthcare technology researcher who had completed similar work in the past.

Furthermore, I had developed a questionnaire for staff and patients about medical device issues. This was designed to provide another data gathering tool to be used with staff and to encourage my interaction with patients, which had happened less often than I would have liked in the first study. I had not talked to patients about their experiences because I had felt awkward disturbing people who were critically ill and receiving treatment. I was allowed to take photos provided that no staff or patients featured in them.

Methodologically, from the first study I concluded the following. (1) It is not practical to get dedicated uninterrupted sit down time with nurses for interviews. Staff were too busy in the Oncology outpatient unit, and after two short interviews were attempted, the manager rejected any more. (2) It is not practical to get written informed consent from patients when you are just work-shadowing staff. Instead, I politely introduced myself to the patient and asked if it was okay to observe the nurse perform the treatment.

3.3   STUDY EXPERIENCE

Since doing the first study in the Oncology outpatient unit I was more familiar with the hospital and staff, e.g., I had met the matron of the Oncology Ward in passing. Consequently, I thought gaining access to it would be relatively quick. This was not the case, and the amount of time to get things completed in healthcare should not be underestimated. It took two weeks to organise a meeting with the Lead Specialist Nurse who has overall responsibility for the wards, a further two weeks to meet the matron who was different from the one I had met before due to staff restructuring, and then a further two weeks to meet the ward manager. All needed to give their permission to allow me on to the ward for the study.

I was apprehensive about my first day. Despite this being the second study, the Oncology ward was still a big change from the Oncology outpatient unit and I was worried about what I might find. Unlike the outpatient unit, patients on wards are likely to be much more unwell and bed ridden. A close friend of mine had passed away due to cancer previously, and some of those memories and emotions were still with me. The ward manager showed me around when I met her to get her permission before the study had started, which was great to acclimatize myself and feel more comfortable, but this was still brief. Being mindful of the challenges in emotionally demanding research, accepting and using emotions in qualitative research, and treating them as a focus of study has been discussed elsewhere (e.g., Gilbert, 2001).

I joined the nurses for their safety briefing. This was at the very start of the shift when all the nurses were together so it was a good opportunity to speak to them all at once. The introduction went well and I distributed the information sheets and consent forms. However, there was a sense of urgency and business that pervaded the whole meeting so the nurses ran off immediately to attend to their patients. I could not get them to sign the consent forms in a rush, and I did not want to delay their work. Instead, I felt it was more important that they understood the main issues, so I briefly highlighted these: that it was a purely voluntary study, any observations would remain anonymous, and I was there to learn as much as possible about medical device use and design.

On subsequent mornings I did not get a chance to introduce myself to the whole group; instead I spoke to the one or two members of staff I had not yet met individually. I came to learn that it was good practice to introduce myself to every member of staff after the safety briefing, regardless of whether I got a general introduction or not, to help break the ice for that day.

From the first study I had learnt that it was important to try to take an apprenticeship stance, as advocated in Contextual Design (Beyer & Holtzblatt, 1998). I got a better response from staff if I was there to "learn from them" rather than "observe them," which seemed more formal and imposing. However, as the study progressed I found that this was not always appropriate. For example, I would need to be an expert when explaining my research and encouraging staff to think that they are not always at fault if a piece of equipment is difficult to use because of its design—an old adage in HCI that can be difficult to grasp if you are completely unfamiliar with it. Furthermore, there was a situation where I felt the need to intervene—beyond what an apprentice stance might comfortably allow—because I was sure a device that was disturbing a patient could be better controlled (described in the oximeter example below).

Soon after I introduced myself, the ward manager instructed me to put my bag and coat in the staff room, as these were not allowed on the ward. Inadvertently this gave me access to the staff common room where I was welcomed to have breaks and lunch too. This invitation never happened in the Oncology outpatient unit as the manager in that situation was keen to protect what little breaks the staff had. After that experience I was keen not to exploit staff breaks for formal data gathering (e.g., interviews) but only in so far as the staff prompted me and it felt comfortable. Here, staff had more time to talk about issues in depth, to consider things, recollect experiences from their past, and talk more freely away from patients and management. They shared information whilst I work-shadowed them too but their attention was often more occupied with the task they were doing. Access to the staff communal spaces was great as it naturally led to me building rapport and gathering extra data, e.g., I quickly found that none of the group knew what a technical feature on the oximeter did and they offered more issues with this device as the conversation developed. It needed sensitivity to protect breaks, e.g., by casually talking about work when invited rather than more purposeful investigation, and this access was not allowed in all situations.

The ward manager showed me around the ward paying particular attention to safety issues, e.g., that I should follow nurses' instructions and avoid rooms that were still radioactive from radiotherapy patients. The ward manager also gave me a tour of their medical devices, describing what they were used for and whether there were any usability issues with them in her opinion. Someone had previously directed me to the electrocardiogram (ECG) machine as a potential area of interest. Apparently, staff often loaded its paper incorrectly. The manager said this was not an issue, which was confirmed by the rest of the staff later. She directed me to the continuous positive airway pressure (CPAP) machine as a potential source of interest as the staff did not like using it. This is a machine that forces air into the patient's lungs using a mask and positive pressure. It was used for patients who have difficulty breathing and low oxygen levels in their blood. The manager introduced me to many other devices—the infusion pumps, hoists, blood glucose monitors, and oximeters, which she thought may be of interest to me but she had not identified any particular problems with their use.

After the manager's introduction and tour, I was left to talk to staff and ask them if I could shadow them when they were using the medical devices. I soon found that everyone was busy and I had no place to conveniently sit or stand where I was out of the way but not too far—so I was not forgotten and could get a feel for what was happening. I had experienced similar in the Oncology outpatient study. The main action seemed to be happening around the clinical area where drugs were prepared, with nurses frequently going in and out, and there was room there so that became my preferred place to hang out, chat and get acclimatised further.

Over the next few study days I found that infusion pumps, which were the main focus of the study, were not used as frequently as I had been led to believe. The staff were confident that they were used frequently but this is not what I found. Many infusions were gravity fed and did not use a pump. Furthermore, I was not around for some infusions—e.g., if they were set up at night, or some infusions were for seriously ill patients which were considered too sensitive for me to observe by some staff, and other infusions were administered when other private activities occurred (e.g., changing a patient's incontinence pads). I did make some infusion pump observations that proved interesting but the length of time I was spending on the ward did not reflect the relatively little data

I was gathering on these devices. Consequently, I sought broader observations on medical devices, and the context, and I looked for interesting data that I could access more frequently.

One device that presented itself as a potentially interesting case where I could gather data more frequently was a new blood glucose meter that had just been introduced to the ward. The healthcare assistants who used this device were happy for me to shadow them on their blood glucose rounds that happen before meal times. This change of research focus gave me data for a thorough evaluation of the device's design and use, and made me feel more confident that I would get something solid out of the time I was spending on the ward.

I was also mindful of other opportunities and leads that might present themselves as interesting areas for study. The CPAP machine was used so infrequently I never saw it set up. I did find a spare one so I could make notes on its design but I never saw it in use. Serendipitously, an interesting situation occurred with an oximeter that I was present for. Previously, the ward manger had introduced the oximeters as non-problematic devices. The oximeters were wheeled up to patients to take their heart rate and blood oxygen saturation levels. These patient spot-checks were frequent. I later found out that the oximeters were also used for continuous monitoring more infrequently. One Saturday morning, a doctor emerged from a patient side room where a device was alarming very loudly. She asked the nurse if there was anything that could be done about the alarm, but the nurse said she had tried everything. When I asked what was happening the nurse explained that the patient was very unwell, had received medication, and his heart rate was very high. The oximeter alarms when the oxygen saturation levels in the blood or the heart rate are too high or low. The nurse said she had tried turning the volume down but it had not worked. I found a spare oximeter to look at; how to turn the volume down was not obvious, even when referring to the instructions printed on top of the device. I found the nurse and asked what she had done. She said she had tried everything. I asked her to show me on the spare one. She pointed to the down arrow. I highlighted the instructions which indicated that the down arrow alone changes the pulse volume, and that to change the alarm volume she should hold the alarm silence button down for at least three seconds and then use the down arrow. She repeated that she had tried everything, but said she would try what I had shown her. The fact the nurse kept saying she had tried everything made me feel that she was not open to suggestions and wanted to appear competent and confident. I got the feeling that she did not want to talk about it as she was very busy with other things too, but I thought the on-going situation with the patient was very sensitive and was sure she would try things to make the situation better. I was clear to point out that the device looked tricky to use, and I also wanted to make sure she did not feel undermined. She asked if I wanted to come in the side room to try, but I declined as I was not allowed to control the devices and the situation had been considered too sensitive for me to attend previously—the patient's wife was in the room comforting him and no one was sure how long he had left. The interaction I suggested did not work either and I later discovered other issues with the device's design and use.

Over the course of the study my perception that some staff were more helpful and engaging than others was reified. In terms of data gathering it can prove productive to recognise "research champions" who will open up opportunities and data that other staff might not. I also learnt to be aware of signs that staff are not keen on taking part, even if they have not directly declined participation in the research. This might be fairly short term if they are having a bad day or longer term for any number of other reasons.

I had never worked night shifts before and found staying awake gruelling to the point I could barely concentrate or think straight. Staff covered for each other whilst they had extended breaks to sleep, although I do not think this was officially approved. I was invited to have a break too and accepted. After taking part in the sleeping breaks I felt more accepted by the staff. Although staff were busy they were concerned with my welfare, e.g., they would ask me to sit down if they thought I had stood for too long and offered me drinks. Long fieldwork days are tiring, but a full 12-h shift from 8 p.m. to 8 a.m. was even harder to complete.

I still never achieved the levels of patient interaction I thought I would. I chatted to patients when shadowing nurses but not for more formal data gathering about their views, including getting informed consent. This is partly because of the awkwardness of disturbing people when they are so unwell, and also because it is hard to know how people are feeling, whether they are drugged or in pain, or whether they can speak English. For example, a student nurse invited me to observe her using a blood pressure machine. As we approached the patient's bed I introduced myself and asked if it was okay if I observe the nurse doing her work as normal. The patient looked at me scared. I explained again saying there was nothing to worry about, but then realised that she could not speak English. I suppose I looked more like a doctor and she probably wondered what I wanted, e.g., "*Was it bad news?*" A more experienced nurse stepped in and made the patient feel at ease—the nurse was cleaning urine from the floor after a patient's accident. The patient did not really want to be confronted with things she did not understand in her state – I can only imagine that if I were asking her to read information sheets and sign forms, it would be worse. It made me think that consent needs to be proportionate to the risks and intrusion the research poses to the patient as formal procedures and signatures could overly worry some patients for what is a brief and trivial interaction.

The more substantial data that I gathered in this study was around the blood glucose meter use because this data was accessible. The infusion pump observations were too infrequent, and the very interesting scenario of the oximeter only happened once. It seems easier to publish on the substantial data I have than the infrequent and interesting events I chanced upon. More recently, a member of staff asked whether my critique of the blood glucose meter was engaging with the real problems of the ward, e.g., when patients in four bed bays are being deprived of sleep because of each other's devices alarming. In a sense it is like the drunk looking for his key under the streetlight; this is where we can gather data most easily and it is harder to publish scientific papers on themes where we have little data. Of course, it may mean we return another time, with a different plan and different resources, to look in those less well lit areas (advice on data gathering can be found in Volume 2: Chapter 4).

3.4   SUMMARY

Different practical, personal, and research experiences are presented in this case study, e.g., in terms of building rapport, data gathering, and research issues. Some provide good topics for debate e.g., what form of consent is appropriate, what strategies are there for interacting with patients comfortably, how do we find focus, and how should we deal with and report learning from infrequent events with little data. These experiences can be shared to facilitate learning. However, there is little substitute for the longer stretches of time needed to mature into this type of work, to learn by doing, and to get a feel for the healthcare domain.

ACKNOWLEDGEMENTS

This work was funded by the CHI+MED project: EPSRC grant EP/G059063/1. Ann Blandford leads the situated interactions research theme within CHI+MED and has supervised me and supported me throughout this work.

CHAPTER 4

Observing Healthcare: An Exploration of Observer Experiences and Emotion

Anjum Chagpar, Svetlena Taneva, Kevin Armour, Cassie McDaniel, Tara McCurdie, Jennifer Jeon, and Deborah Chan

This chapter describes the collective experiences of the authors based on fieldwork studies in the magnetic resonance imaging, radiation therapy, and surgical domains. In exploring the authors' emotional reactions to what they encounter during fieldwork, it attempts to prime those who are new to shadowing in healthcare, to situations they may find themselves in. Specifically, this chapter looks at the emotions of a researcher when faced with:

- Learning of a patient's life-changing diagnosis, before the patient herself;

- Realising your presence in the clinical setting is a factor that poses a serious risk to patient safety; and

- Seeing only a fragment from a patient's critical illness journey and not knowing the patient's health outcome.

4.1 INTRODUCTION

Those of us conducting fieldwork in healthcare not only need to be prepared for the logistical and ethical complexities of shadowing in clinical environments, but also for our own emotional reactions to the experience of observing. In healthcare, this often means observing those in compromised physical and emotional states. It means observing safety-critical procedures with potentially life-altering consequences. And as outsiders, it often means knowing only part of what happens to the people we are observing. This chapter describes the collective experiences of the authors based on fieldwork studies in the magnetic resonance imaging (MRI), radiation therapy, and surgical domains, and the strong emotional reactions in those conducting the observations. This complements the section on emotion in Volume 2: Chapter 2.

4.2   STUDY DESIGN

Much of the fieldwork described in the stories that follow aims to understand current clinical practices and technologies with the goal of improving their safety and efficiency. Specifically, when shadowing in MRI suites, our goal was to identify ways to optimise interfaces and processes in order to streamline workflow. While shadowing radiation therapists, we sought to understand the challenges faced by clinicians using complex software to deliver powerful radiation beams to cancer patients, and use this knowledge to design improved interfaces (Chan et al., 2010). Finally, we observed a number of surgeries as part of a project to procure an optimal Anesthesia Information System for the 18 Operating Rooms (ORs) at a large academic health sciences centre.

4.3   OBSERVATION EXPERIENCES

The stories below are first person accounts of fieldwork experiences that were common to our group, despite the diverse domains and environments studied. Taken together, these stories reveal common lessons that have benefited all members of our team when observing.

4.3.1   OBSERVING THE VULNERABLE

From Kevin Armour: My first experience performing ethnographic research in the medical field focused on understanding the workflow and software interaction in an MRI unit. As an industrial designer, I was comfortable conducting ethnographic research, as it is a main component of the design process, but all my previous experience had been with consumer products.

I was seated in the control room, conducting interviews with the technicians between patient scans. My initial attention was centred on the interface and noting various layouts and workflow constraints when the first patient was brought into the imaging room alone, visibly nervous, and set up on the MRI table for imaging. As her image appeared on the screen, I was struck by the details of her physical anatomy that I was able to see. She had a large growth in her abdomen, which the technician commented was in fact cancerous. When the imaging was complete, the patient was helped off the table and brought through the control room. She asked the technician about what he may or may not have seen, seeking reassurance, and scanned our faces to see if she could infer the results. The technician informed her that the images first needed to be reviewed by her physicians before a diagnosis could be made.

In that moment, I knew that this patient's life would be changing dramatically. I knew she would not receive the reassurance that she was hoping for. And I knew she was frightened by this scan and would likely have many more scans ahead of her. Knowing so much more than she did left me feeling like my presence had compromised both her dignity and privacy.

While I would certainly respect her privacy and not disclose what I saw in any identifiable way, I would always know what I saw. In effect, did my presence not compromise her privacy?

4.3.2 OBSERVING THE DANGEROUS

From Svetlena Taneva: While conducting fieldwork in a radiation therapy unit of a large teaching hospital, I was sitting in the control area with the radiation therapists (RTs) whom I had interviewed prior to a patient's treatment. Radiation delivery began. This is a safety-critical time when RTs monitor the patient in the treatment room via a camera, as well as watch the control software for status and error messages. During beam delivery, one of the RTs was eager to continue sharing insights about his work. As he was speaking to me, he was illustrating some of his points about the radiation therapy software by switching screens and clicking on different options. While he did not seem concerned about engaging in these tasks, I became aware that my presence had become a distraction. I was also well aware of the risks that distractions introduce in the context of safety-critical tasks. In addition, I was familiar with radiation therapy incident reports where patients had received enormous amounts of radiation and died due to overdoses because the RTs had not monitored the camera and software screens. My discomfort was compounded by the fact that in his desire to help out in my study, the RT was switching screens and clicking on software options while the patient was receiving radiation. I politely told the RT that we could resume after the patient's treatment was finished, but he said he did not mind discussing the issues and continued. I was not sure how to tactfully insist on pausing the conversation and so I continued listening while a number of frightening thoughts crossed my mind. Thankfully, no incidents occurred!

This experience changed the way I see my role professionally while *in situ*. It has also changed the way I will experience healthcare in my personal life, as a patient—knowing that clinicians can lack awareness of their cognitive limitations as related to multi-tasking, distractions, and interruptions during safety-critical tasks will make me an apprehensive and nervous patient.

4.3.3 OBSERVING THE INCOMPLETE

From Anjum Chagpar: One of my first field studies was aimed at understanding anaesthesiology workflow, tasks, and environments. I observed several anaesthesiologists before, during, and after, surgical procedures. As it became clear that most of the work complexity occurred in the ORs, I began to focus my observations there. Often I arrived as the patient was being prepped for surgery. In the pre-operative clinic, the patient and their family members would meet with members of the surgical team and talk about the process and any concerns. Shortly after, the patient would be wheeled into the OR and sedated before the surgery began. Because I was shadowing in a tertiary academic hospital, many of the procedures performed were complex, and took several hours to complete. As a result, I often left the OR before the surgery was finished. After conducting several shadowing sessions in which I watched the patient undergo sedation, and left before they were brought back to consciousness, I began to feel a sense of unease around shadowing. It was not until I observed a complete procedure, including watching the patient wake up in the post-operative recovery area, that I realised why. My initial introductions to the patients were optimistic and warm, but my final observations were of unconscious, exposed, and powerless bodies, nothing like the people whom I had met a few hours earlier. It was this disparity between my first and last experiences of the patients that were causing me to feel so uncomfortable.

While I was not conscious of it at first, I had formed emotional attachments to the patients I was observing. I wanted a good outcome for them, and at the very least, to know what happened to them. In the case of the surgery patients, I wanted to see them awake and surrounded by family as they were when I first met them. But the reality of observing healthcare often means we are only able to experience a part of the patient's story. How do we deal with the lack of closure, uncertainty, and questions that remain?

4.4   LESSONS LEARNED

4.4.1   THERE IS NO SUCH THING AS A FLY ON THE WALL

When conducting fieldwork in healthcare, it is common to see patients in extremely vulnerable states: undressed, emotionally distraught or undergoing life-threatening procedures. The fact that we are physically present, especially in constrained spaces, in and of itself, can change the dynamic of what we are observing. In addition, because we cannot un-know what we have seen, patient privacy may in fact be compromised. For example, being present when a cancer diagnosis is revealed to a patient means that there is one additional person who knows this information, who would not have otherwise. Our presence may change the patient's response compared to if we were not there. This Hawthorne effect is well known, and as observers we are taught to minimize the bias it introduces (Monahan & Fisher, 2010). Yet behaving as if we are not present in these vulnerable situations can sometimes compromise our own sense of humanity, leading us to feel uncomfortable and disconnected. Accepting the reality that our presence can and does impact what we are observing can lead to a willingness to demonstrate compassion and express concern during our fieldwork.

4.4.2   THERE IS NO SUCH THING AS A NAÏVE OBSERVER

Because we are human, and have our own and our loved ones' health to consider, each of us has a vested interest when observing healthcare situations. Our experiences and our biases shape how we react to what we are observing at the moment, as well as how we will behave in the future. In particular, as human factors professionals working in healthcare, we are acutely aware of process inefficiencies, safety issues and human cognitive limitations. While on the one hand we do not want to be perceived as auditors or evaluators, there are times when as observers we may need to share our experiences and knowledge. At the same time, we must also be aware that our presence may be a distraction that further contributes to the issues being observed. As researchers, we ourselves are the instruments of measurement, and must be aware of the role our own histories play in what we are observing (advice on data gathering and reflexivity can be found in Volume 2).

4.4.3 SHARING STORIES HELPS

It is surprising how little time it takes to become emotionally invested in someone you have never met after observing them in a vulnerable situation. Because we are not clinicians, and are not responsible for the care of the patients we are observing, it is easy to feel powerless when we see people suffering. While the reality of patient ethics and privacy means that we often do not have the opportunity to learn what the final outcomes are for the people we have observed, we have found that collectively we have experiences to draw upon which may help close the loop (Hedican, 2006).

Sharing stories with others who have experienced parts of patient journeys that you have not can provide some boundaries around the open question of *"what happened to that person?"* So while the opportunity to know first hand may not be available, envisioning a specific positive outcome may be easier based on this shared knowledge of possible outcomes. In effect, this envisioning equates to a directed wish for the best for the person you observed, which for many of us, speaks to why we have entered into the healthcare domain in the first place.

ACKNOWLEDGEMENT

The authors wish to thank the clinicians and patients who graciously consented to being observed for our studies.

CHAPTER 5

Finding Balance: Matters of Ethics, Consent, and Emotional Work When Studying Handover in Hospitals

Rebecca Randell

This chapter recounts the experience of undertaking fieldwork across a range of hospital settings as part of a three-year project that developed a model of handover to inform technology design. The specific issues addressed in this chapter are:

- The challenges of consenting patients who are in distressing situations;

- The feelings and images that stay with us after we leave the clinical setting; and

- The need to find balance among multiple priorities: ethics, research, researcher, data collection time, fieldnotes, and analysis.

5.1 RESEARCH FOCUS

Handover is a process that involves the passing and acceptance of responsibility for some or all aspects of care for a patient, or group of patients, and the sharing of relevant information (Wilson et al., 2009). Shift handovers and transfers are both regular features of hospital work, shift handovers taking place between oncoming and outgoing staff when there is a shift change and transfers occurring when a patient is moved from one ward or hospital to another.

Successful handover is essential for patient safety (Junior Doctors Committee, 2004). Handovers have become more frequent, due to shorter working hours for doctors, a result of regulations such as the European Working Time Directive, and due to greater specialisation in medicine which has led to an increase in patients being transferred between wards and hospitals.

The importance of handover for patient safety, combined with the increased frequency, has led to interest in providing technological support for handover (Junior Doctors Committee, 2004). GHandI (Generic Handover Investigation) was a three-year project that, through data collection across a range of hospital settings, developed a model of handover to inform technology design (Randell et al., 2011a, 2011b; Randell et al., 2010, 2011).

In this chapter, I reflect on my experience of undertaking that data collection. Rather than giving a general account of my experience, I have chosen to focus on two key topics—consenting patients and the broader emotional challenges—so as to be able to explore these topics in greater depth.

5.2 STUDY DESIGN

A multi-site case study design, with ethnographic observation, was used (Yin, 2003). We anticipated collecting data from ten case sites. In practice, we carried out observations in eight sites, spread across four National Health Service (NHS) hospitals in the south east of England: an emergency assessment unit (EAU), a general medical ward, a medical assessment unit (MAU), a high dependency unit (HDU), a paediatric acute retrieval service (PARS), a paediatric intensive care unit (PICU), a postnatal ward, and a paediatric surgical ward. Interviews were conducted with a ninth site.

Five of the eight sites were ones where we had originally planned to carry out data collection. The other three sites were opportunities that arose once data collection had begun. The MAU and HDU were at a hospital where technology to support handover was being introduced and, through personal contacts at that hospital who were aware of the project, we were invited to participate in the evaluation of the technology. We were introduced to staff at the PICU by the PARS so that we could develop and evaluate technology to support handovers from the PARS to the PICU. One of the sites that had agreed to be part of the study, a PICU in a different hospital, withdrew because they felt that the methods for consenting patients were not appropriate for their setting (discussed further below).

Data collection was conducted predominantly by myself, with another researcher assisting, particularly in the early stages of the research. We aimed to spend approximately three weeks in each case site and to observe a range of types of handovers (shift handovers and transfers) with variation in participants (medical, nursing, allied health professionals). While our focus was on handover, we also wanted to understand the broader work practices and methods for sharing information within each setting. In practice, the amount of time spent in each site varied. We spent 172 h over 14 days observing in the first case site as we came to understand the process of handover, with less time being spent in subsequent settings (typically around 100 h over approximately 10 days per site). The data was collected between May 2007 and October 2009.

5.3 STUDY EXPERIENCE

5.3.1 GAINING CONSENT

Where possible, we wanted to audio-record the handovers but we required written consent from both the staff and the patients to do this. The experience of gaining consent varied according to the setting and the type of handover. For example, in the paediatric surgical ward and the general medical ward, the pace of work and the infrequency of transfers meant that there was adequate time to gain consent from the necessary people. However, in settings where patients were frequently transferred, such as the EAU and MAU, a lot of time was taken up with the process of gaining consent as new patients arrived on the ward, distracting from the task of data collection.

With the PARS, who picked up critically ill children from paediatric HDUs in the south east of England to take them to PICUs in London, gaining consent meant approaching parents who had just learned that their child was critically ill. While all parents consented, and most were happy to talk, I felt uncomfortable with approaching them at that time and questioned the ethics of it and whether it could really be considered "informed consent" when their thoughts were so concerned with other matters. It was also difficult to get consent from the staff in the units that the children were collected from and taken to; while often the PARS team would introduce me to staff, on other occasions there was not time for such introductions.

Similarly, although not a distressing situation, in the postnatal ward I often felt uncomfortable approaching the mothers for consent. Not only were they typically exhausted, but I also felt that I was intruding on an intimate moment as they and their partner got to know their new baby. More generally, across the settings, I had to manage the conflict between the need to obtain consent while not wanting to impose. For some patients, the effort of reading the information sheet was too much. While most patients were happy to take part, I sometimes felt it was as a favour to me rather than due to their interest in the project.

The PICU that withdrew from the project did so because they felt that our process for consenting patients was unworkable in their setting. They wanted us to have an opt-out consent process, where notices would be put up around the unit and patients and their families could say if they did not want to be included in the study. The postnatal ward said that they would also prefer an opt-out consent process. We submitted an amendment to the NHS ethics committee, requesting to change our consent process for these two sites, but the amendment was not approved. However, the postnatal ward were still happy to participate in the study.

5.3.2 STRESSES AND STRAINS OF FIELDWORK

In undertaking the fieldwork, I worked long, antisocial hours, including some weekends and the occasional night shift. If I wanted to observe the nurses' morning handover at 7 a.m., I would need to get to the hospital before then, to see the preparation that was made before the handover. One of the hospitals where we conducted observations was some distance from my home and so this required me to get up at 5 a.m. On numerous occasions, I stayed at the hospital from before the morning handover until after the evening handover.

Not only was the fieldwork physically tiring, I also found it emotionally tiring. One of my clearest memories is of crying in a hospital car park after learning that a child who had been on the paediatric surgical ward had died from a hospital-acquired infection after being transferred to her local hospital. This was a child who I had spent time playing with while undertaking fieldwork in the ward. While the nurses had their own practices for responding to these events, I was excluded from these practices but also, as a researcher, I felt that I had less right to be upset than those nurses who had cared for her. There are a range of other images that stick in my mind, despite the years that have passed: the elderly patient repeatedly crying out that she wanted to die, the critically ill baby, the man who wanted to be discharged because he did not want his wife to worry. When I think of these moments, what I am reminded of is the feelings that pervaded the atmosphere: distress, anxiety, and sadness.

Even without the long hours and without the distressing situations, the stresses of fieldwork are well acknowledged (Hammersley & Atkinson, 1995). When you enter the field, you are entering an unfamiliar environment, and with this study it was a process I had to repeatedly go through. This is an essential part of fieldwork; Hammersley and Atkinson (1995) describe the comfortable sense of being "at home" as a danger signal, that there is not the necessary social and intellectual distance needed for a critical perspective. I have other images, which remind me of the strangeness of the situations I found myself in: sat in the front of an ambulance, driving fast down the hard shoulder of the motorway or on the wrong side of the road during London rush hour; seeing a prisoner in handcuffs being escorted through the hospital by police officers; a woman who gave birth not having realised she was pregnant.

One of the first challenges in a number of the settings was trying to track down the medical handovers and the attendant fear of not being able to get the necessary data. Medical handovers sometimes took place in corridors or cafes, so gaining access to such handovers required me to either shadow the people whose handovers I wanted to observe or to quickly build up adequate rapport so that they would inform me when and where the handover would take place. Building and maintaining such relationships could also be tiring, repeatedly explaining and justifying my presence. As with all fieldwork, the research required me to always be alert, both for the purposes of the research but also to be sensitive to the situation, managing the conflict between the need and desire to gather data while not wanting to get in the way.

Fieldwork can affect us in ways that are hard to anticipate. The long hours, the lone working, and the tiring nature of the work meant that I had less contact with my usual network of support. I found that spending long hours on hospital wards pushed my thoughts in a particular direction, to reflect on my own mortality and to consider how I would respond if I or someone close to me was in such a situation. I also think that the large amount of fieldwork led, at times, to a feeling of saturation where I lost my inquisitiveness because I felt that I had heard it all before (Hammersley & Atkinson, 1995).

5.4   REFLECTIONS

Despite the challenges described above, I enjoy doing fieldwork; I feel privileged to get to understand other people's working environments in that way, while most people only know their own working environment. I continue to do fieldwork because that is the only way we truly understand the detail of how that work takes place. I could have chosen to research a different kind of environment but I have stayed with healthcare in the hope that my research can lead to improvements in patient care.

However, there are things that we can do to make fieldwork in healthcare settings a better experience for the researcher, most of which are a question of balance.

5.4.1   BALANCING THE DEMANDS OF ETHICS COMMITTEES WITH THE DEMANDS OF THE RESEARCH

Firstly, it is necessary to balance the demands of ethics committees with the demands of the research. Rather than coming up with a process that will please the ethics committee but which then gets in the way of doing the research, it is necessary to come up with processes that are feasible and then make a clear argument to the ethics committee about why the proposed processes are appropriate. This requires talking with healthcare professionals within the settings and may mean that it is necessary to have different processes of consent for different settings. You could also establish a "patient panel," of people who have experience as patients in the types of settings you are interested in, and get their perspective on appropriate processes. Such consultation with healthcare professionals and patients will also demonstrate to the ethics committee that you have thought through what you are going to do.

In the U.K., for the meantime at least, NHS ethical approval is no longer necessary for research that just involves NHS staff, a change that is likely to help many HCI researchers doing this kind of work. I think it helps to be clear about what information we want to gather and for what purpose, because in most cases we are not interested in patient identifiable information. More recently, I submitted an ethics application to video record multidisciplinary team meetings. It would have been impractical to obtain consent from patients for this but I explained that we were not interested in patient identifiable information, instead being interested in the types of information that were communicated, and that no patient identifiable information would be transcribed. This was approved without question.

Those in the setting, and patient representatives, can also give feedback on information sheets and consent forms. Taking the time to design information sheets and consent forms which are easy to understand, explaining the purpose of the research in everyday language which makes clear the intended outcomes of the research, can ease the process of seeking consent once fieldwork begins.

5.4.2   BALANCING THE NEEDS OF THE RESEARCH WITH THE NEEDS OF THE RESEARCHER

Secondly, it is necessary to balance the needs of the research with the needs of the researcher. When I look back at the study protocol, although I had written details of what data we wanted to collect and talked about observing on different days of the week and at different times of day, there was no clear plan of what hours would be spent doing this. There is a need to get away from the romantic notion of the lone ethnographer and think practically about what is manageable, acknowledging that fieldwork is tiring (see Volume 2: Chapter 2 for advice on how you can prepare yourself for undertaking fieldwork).

The researcher has to manage their fear of "missing something." While it was interesting to see how the information communicated at the beginning of the shift had changed over the course of the day, after observing for 13 h writing up my fieldnotes was not my first priority and it could be argued that having more accurate and vivid fieldnotes is more important than trying to capture everything. Where possible, having two researchers working together is a good idea, so that they can support each other and reflect on their experiences together. It also means that, when there is a desire to capture developments over time, this can be shared between the two researchers.

5.4.3   BALANCING TIME FOR DATA COLLECTION WITH TIME FOR ANALYSIS

This ties in with my third point, which concerns balancing time for data collection with time for writing up fieldnotes and analysing the data. A clear plan for data collection should schedule in time for writing up fieldnotes, ideally as soon after observation as possible. The more time goes by before fieldnotes are written up, the less vivid your memories will be, making it harder to fill in the contextual details that are missing from your "jottings" (Emerson et al., 1995) in the field. A strategy that may be useful, when the nature of the fieldwork prevents writing up fieldnotes straight away, is to dictate your fieldnotes at the end of day, for later transcription (McDonald, 2005; see also Volume 2: Chapter 4 for suggestions of other sources of data that can supplement your fieldnotes, such as photographs of the setting). Writing up fieldnotes should not be rushed, allowing for reflection that can inform subsequent data collection. As a rough rule of thumb, 1 h for writing up fieldnotes should be allowed for each hour of data collection (Emerson et al., 1995).

GHandI was ambitious in its intention to study ten different settings and while that ambition is admirable and I believe strongly in the need for multi-site studies in HCI in order to come up with more generalizable findings, it is a lot for one or two researchers to undertake. We collected a huge amount of data and, while all of it was analysed, I think that we could have learnt much more from that data if we had more time for analysis.

There is no consensus regarding how many case sites to include in a multi-site case study. The number of case sites depends on the number of aspects of the context that are anticipated to impact on the phenomenon of interest (Yin, 2003), while also involving a trade-off between breadth and depth of investigation (Hammersley & Atkinson, 1995). In my experience, four case sites is a manageable amount, enabling identification of organisational level factors that impact the phenomenon of interest while providing confidence in the generalizability of findings that are consistent across sites (Dowding et al., 2009). Alternatively, theoretical sampling could be used, where the researcher takes an iterative approach to data collection and analysis and uses the emerging theory to select new settings, stopping when data saturation is reached (Glaser & Strauss, 1967). Limiting the amount of data collection in this way, and having adequate breaks between periods of fieldwork, can also reduce feelings of overload.

ACKNOWLEDGEMENT

This work was funded by the U.K. Engineering and Physical Sciences Research Council (EPSRC) through the GHandI project (grant number EP/D078636/1).

CHAPTER 6

Fieldwork and Challenges of Access

Brian Hilligoss

This case study explores challenges encountered while conducting a two-year ethnographic study of doctors' admissions work in a highly specialised U.S. academic medical centre. The particular issues discussed in this chapter are:

- How to gain access to a research site;

- Difficulties with approaching multiple professions within the healthcare setting; and

- Gaining access to patient data.

6.1   RESEARCH FOCUS

I study the communication and coordination processes entailed in interdependent organisational routines in healthcare settings. My research is driven by a desire to understand the relationships between organisational structures and the collective actions of healthcare workers. The structures I study include information and communication technologies, culture, routines, hierarchies, and divisions of labour. Much of my work is couched in larger discourses aimed at understanding and improving the quality and safety of healthcare delivery systems.

One frequently repeated and highly important clinical communication and coordination activity is the patient handoff (also referred to as handover): *"the exchange between health professionals of information about a patient accompanying either a transfer of control over, or of responsibility for, the patient"* (Cohen & Hilligoss, 2010). In recent years, many have grown increasingly concerned that handoffs may compromise patient safety (Beach et al., 2003) and negatively impact quality of care (Behara et al., 2005; Horwitz et al., 2009). However, further research is needed, including that which deepens our understanding of handoff practice as it occurs in the field (Wears, 2012). Randell (this volume: Chapter 5) also discusses lessons from studying handoffs to inform technology design.

6.2   STUDY DESIGN

Between January 2009 and March 2011, I conducted an ethnographic study of doctors' admissions work at Memorial Hospital (a pseudonym), an adult acute care, and a highly specialised tertiary academic medical centre located in the United States. My aim was to understand the challenges entailed in admissions work, particularly in handing off responsibility from the Emergency Department (ED) to various inpatient units, including both internal medicine and surgical services, when patients are admitted to the hospital. I used a constructivist Grounded Theory approach (Charmaz, 2006) since my goal was to refine how handoffs are conceptualized and to construct a substantive theoretical explanation for handoff practice variation.

A total of 86 individuals participated, including both residents (i.e., house officers) and attending doctors and several hospital administrators. Since most of my work focused on the transition between the ED and General Internal Medicine services, including both resident and hospitalist services, most of my participants were physicians working in these units.

Between January 2009 and June 2010, I conducted a total of 349 h of field observations. These were roughly divided between the ED and the general medicine hospitalist and resident services. Observations ranged in duration from three to eight hours and entailed shadowing and interacting with either a resident or an attending doctor engaged in admissions work. I did not directly participate in clinical activities. I carried a small notebook with me and took brief notes. At the end of each day, I typed up these notes, elaborating from memory. I also conducted 48 semi-structured interviews with doctors on various services, as well as numerous brief informal interviews with various personnel during the course of my observations.

6.3   STUDY EXPERIENCE

I frame the discussion of my experiences as challenges of access. Here, I explore three: challenges of gaining (1) access to a site, (2) access to different perspectives, and (3) access to patient data. For a discussion of access issues more generally, see Volume 2: Chapter 3.

6.3.1   ACCESS TO A SITE

In fieldwork we often have to begin wherever we find an open door. Access can be difficult for the outsider to acquire generally, but especially to hospitals. A doctoral student at the time I started this project, I was fortunate in that my advisor had already forged a collegial relationship with and introduced me to someone influential within the hospital. This individual introduced me to several heads of units within the hospital via email. At the same time, I met another doctoral student who had completed some work with a senior physician administrator in the ED. This doctoral student very helpfully introduced me to that individual. These connections opened doors for me, leading to invitations to interview and observe in multiple units. I very much doubt that I would have found such welcome access—at least not so quickly—had it not been for the reputations and help of these individuals.

The obvious lesson here is the importance of networking to securing access. Why should people open up their work to the close observation of complete strangers? The reality is they often will not, so the connections of others with respected reputations are invaluable. To build our networks, we should always be reaching out, meeting new people, sharing our interests, and inquiring about theirs.

The connection of my doctoral student friend to the ED administrator led to my meeting in person with the latter. As it turned out, he had an existing interest in improving the quality of handoffs in his unit and, thus, welcomed my request to observe. Another vital takeaway is that we need to demonstrate the relevance of our proposed research to those whose work and environment we hope to study. They have every right to ask, "*What's in it for me?*" Part of our chore, then, is to understand their problems, challenges, and concerns and to look for ways to help address these as we simultaneously pursue our own agendas. A good starting place for any fieldwork is understanding what concerns and challenges people in the setting perceive relevant to the issues we want to study (Van de Ven, 2007). This not only helps orient us to the phenomenon, it also provides us insight into what we need to keep in mind as the study progresses if we are to have a practical impact in the immediate setting.

6.3.2   ACCESS TO DIFFERENT PERSPECTIVES

Tertiary academic medical centres are large, complex organisations. Work in these settings is subdivided across many different individuals, professions, specialties, and administrative units, heavily dependent on myriad technologies. Such a complex system can look very different depending on the perspective from which one is viewing it. Developing a nuanced understanding of work requires examining it from multiple perspectives. For me, this proved challenging.

Largely out of a desire to manage scope, I decided early on to focus my study on the work of doctors and the handoffs between them. I suppose I focused on doctors because the initial doors that opened to me provided me direct access to doctors. Perhaps if my initial contacts had been nurses, my study might have ultimately been focused on that profession. Nurses also play an important role in admissions work and have their own handoff processes that happen in parallel with doctors' handoffs. But the work of nurses and doctors seemed sufficiently distinct that I felt justified in focusing on doctors. At some point during my observations, however, I began to realise that actions of doctors had consequences for the work of nurses and that, likewise, actions of nurses could have consequences for the work of doctors. To develop a richer understanding of doctors' admissions work, it seemed potentially useful to interview some nurses. Surprisingly, this proved to be a nearly impossible challenge for me.

After spending several months observing in the ED, I mentioned to my primary contact there (the physician administrator) that I thought I might benefit from talking to some nurses. I could observe them as they worked in the ED, but observing them did not give me access to their thinking and perspectives. My contact put me in touch via email with the chief charge nurse for the ED. Over the course of several months—yes, months—through a series of emails, I tried to arrange a meeting with the charge nurse and to come up with a plan for focus groups with nurses. Although occasionally it seemed I was making progress, there was always someone else the charge nurse needed to speak to or clear some detail with. The email exchange would fall silent. I would write to inquire on progress: no answer. I would write again, several times, before I would get an answer. Most ideas I proposed were eventually shot down as not possible. The charge nurse very much doubted that nurses would voluntarily give up their own time to attend interviews or focus groups. I offered to provide gift cards as incentives for participation (I had a small research fund). After a few months I was told Human Resources would not allow this—something about union regulations. I offered to provide a lunch. This was met with concerns that it would not be fair to the other nurses. I eventually met some very senior nurse administrators in the hospital and asked their advice. They promised to help, but little came of this as well. Frustrated, I eventually gave up.

At some point in the process, I began to wonder if the seeming resistance I was experiencing from nursing stemmed from the fact I started with doctors. I will never know for certain, but the idea highlights an on-going challenge when doing fieldwork in a setting where a diverse group of professionals work more or less in shared spaces. How do I, as the fieldworker, remain sufficiently neutral to attain necessary access to a diversity of perspectives? Had I inadvertently sent a message that I was "in" with the doctors, and therefore, positioned myself squarely on one side of the doctor-nurse divide? Related, more than once, while observing, I had a nurse or technician make a comment to me—sometimes in a humorous way—that implied they thought I might be evaluating them. A man, standing by watching, not doing anything, can certainly appear to be some sort of evaluator. I always attempted to immediately correct these impressions by stressing that I was studying organisational processes, not people, and that I was a student not an administrator. Of course, it is impossible to say how well I convinced these questioning parties.

This brings up the issue of what the fieldworker wears while observing. There is no right answer to this question in my view. It depends on one's objectives and the particulars of the setting. But, the important point is that appearance probably does matter. Early on in my observations I showed up dressed much the way the attending physicians I was observing were dressed: in a conservative dress shirt and tie, dress pants or khakis, and dark-coloured comfortable shoes. Eventually, I began observing ED residents, who were typically dressed in scrubs, and began to question my clothing choices. Should I omit the tie? Sometimes I did, but since attendings were always nearby in the ED, other times I did not.

On the inpatient side, I fell into a particular pattern. When observing hospitalists, who always wore more professional, business-like attire, I wore a tie. When observing on-call residents—those who were responsible for taking admissions—I omitted the tie and also wore khakis since these residents were nearly always in scrubs and no attendings were around. More than once someone offered to give me a white coat to wear. I refused. My thinking: that was a symbol of being a doctor, including having a particular knowledgebase, expertise, and status that I not only did not have, but did not want anyone to think I had. I felt that maintaining my image as a social scientist and doctoral student was important if I were to appear non-threatening. By the same token, I felt I should present myself such that I looked enough like a doctor that they would respect me and open up to me.

Even in studying doctors I had to navigate professional divisions. Surgeons, internal medicine physicians, and emergency medicine physicians are importantly distinct professional groups, to say nothing of sub-specialists within each of these larger specialties. As it turned out, there were significant, on-going debates among these different specialties pertaining to admissions and the appropriate placement of patients on various services. Surgeons resisted taking admissions of patients who had medical comorbidities that might complicate surgeries, while internal medicine physicians felt patients who came to the hospital for a problem that was *surgical in nature* should be admitted to surgery. Sub-specialists and generalists debated whether a given patient was sufficiently acute or complicated to require sub-specialty care. Surgeons and internal medicine doctors often felt ED physicians were too conservative and admitted patients who could be sent home, while ED physicians felt that doctors on inpatient services sometimes tried to avoid work. These debates were fascinating to me as someone who studies organisational behaviour, but presented a challenge for me as a fieldworker. To fully understand the complexities behind these debates, I needed to examine them from all angles, but to do so, I had to maintain sufficient neutrality so that individuals would be comfortable opening up and sharing their thoughts freely.

To maintain this neutral position, I spent time observing in both the ED and general internal medicine services. By alternating between the two departments, I avoided "going native" and seeing the phenomenon from one perspective or getting sucked into one or the other side of the on-going debates. Furthermore, by studying the phenomenon from both sides, I was able to use what I was learning from my observations in one unit to guide my observations in the other and to generate questions to probe for richer data. For example, some ED physicians viewed pushback from internal medicine doctors as attempts to avoid work. Had I studied the phenomenon only from observations in the ED, I might have accepted this explanation more or less unreservedly. By pairing my ED observations with observations in internal medicine services, however, I came to understand much of this pushback as motivated by genuine concerns about safety and appropriate use of services. Ultimately, this complicated my understanding of the setting and phenomena and moved me to look more deeply for organisational structures and processes that might be contributing to the dynamic I was witnessing.

6.3.3   ACCESS TO PATIENT DATA

Because my focus was on doctor-doctor communication and efforts to coordinate care among these providers, I never attempted to gain direct access to patients. When doctors I was shadowing went into patient rooms, I waited in the hallway, observing the pulse and flow of activity that made up the general context. I relied on summaries from doctors to learn something about their interactions with patients. I did however think that there might be value in looking at patient records in the electronic medical record (EMR), to compare, for instance, how doctors described patients in hand-offs with how they described those same patients in the notes they wrote in their charts. I, therefore, requested permission to access the charts of those patients whose ED admission handoffs I had observed. Although I had to talk to a number of people before I finally found the office with the authority to grant me such access, the overall process was fairly simple. It took several months to get permission from both the hospital and the Institutional Review Board (IRB), but I was granted access to the hospital's EMR.

That lasted about two months. One day I received a call from the IRB notifying me that I should discontinue accessing the EMR. The hospital, in conjunction with the IRB, had unilaterally rescinded all access to patient records for research purposes over concerns that access had been granted inconsistently. No further access was to be permitted until a new policy could be put in place. Months passed. My observations continued, but no further information regarding access to the EMR came. Eventually, I accepted that that portion of my research would have to be abandoned if I was to finish the work on schedule. Fortunately, examining patient records had never been central to my research question, so the effect was minimal. I had more than enough data, but I had lost one additional dimension. For me the lesson in this is the need for flexibility where access to patient data is concerned. In general, most places are still trying to find the right balance between providing access for research purposes and protecting patient privacy. The rescinding of access was abrupt. I never anticipated it nor was given any indication that it was a possibility (other than in the event of any misconduct, of course). For studies where access to patient data is crucial, researchers must be prepared for such events, particularly if individual informed consent is not solicited.

6.4   CONCLUSION

Gaining access—to sites, to perspectives, to data—is a common challenge to most types of fieldwork, no less so in healthcare settings. Long-standing divides between professions, differing approaches to care and treatment among specialisations, hierarchical power structures, and sensitivities about privacy, malpractice, and other such concerns all converge to slow or even prevent the fieldworker's entry. And yet, the complexity implied by these various barriers directly speaks to the tremendous need for fieldwork, for it is the complex environment or process that most demands the deep understanding that only ethnographic approaches provide if needed improvements are to be made.

The lessons I offer from my own experiences seeking access in healthcare settings are these. Cultivate your network. Seek to understand and incorporate into your research the problems of concern to the people you study. Get close but keep your distance, and by that I mean that you need to be close enough to earn the confidence of individuals but distant enough so that their rivals will also trust you. What you wear and how you look probably matters. Expect surprises: some may be fortuitous, but some almost certainly will not. And so, above all, be flexible.

ACKNOWLEDGEMENT

This work was supported by grant number R36HS018758 from the U.S. Agency for Healthcare Research and Quality. The content is solely the responsibility of the author and does not necessarily represent the official views of the Agency for Healthcare Research and Quality.

CHAPTER 7

Building Relationships: HCI Researchers at a Gastro Surgical Department

Kristina Groth and Oscar Frykholm

As healthcare technology researchers, we have conducted fieldwork at a gastrointestinal surgical department, responsible for the upper abdominal tract, during over a period of five years. The first two years focused on being in the field, observing different activities, meetings, and talking to people in order to learn about the setting. The last three years focused on cooperative design methods while developing a decision support system. Three points of focus from this case study are:

- The serendipitous events that led to the start of this fruitful and long-term collaboration;

- The development and maintenance of the close working relationship we had with the healthcare staff at the gastro surgical department; and

- The challenges of working in this area, e.g., we found it difficult to make long-term planning in order to fit into the physicians' schedules and the availability of a test environment would have been a benefit.

7.1 RESEARCH FOCUS

Medical decision-making is an increasingly complex task that involves a number of medical specialisations and technologies. This has led to a growing trend of organising staff in multi-disciplinary teams (Ruhstaller et al., 2006). Our work focuses on a team activity where physicians of different specialisations coordinate and discuss the results of their specific examinations in order to decide on further treatment of the patient: a so-called multidisciplinary team meeting (MDTM). This kind of team-based care is necessary for making the best judgment of a patient's condition, disease, and treatment.

Our study of highly specialised care at a gastro surgical department (hereafter named Gastro) at Karolinska University Hospital in Stockholm, Sweden, has focused on the use of two organisational tools; a network-based care chain and video mediated MDTMs. The care chain was created in order to manage coordination between individuals with different expertise that are distributed at different departments and hospitals, as well as a need to collaborate on tasks that must be completed with fairly strict deadlines. The use of MDTMs has become an important work process in cancer-related healthcare (Kane et al., 2011). In such meetings, a number of medical specialists present and discuss available patient information that is based on, for instance, examinations, previous treatments, lab results, and meetings with the patient.

Technology support in healthcare poses special difficulties, as it must attend to different roles and settings, as well as to patient safety issues. Communication failures have been identified as a common cause of error in healthcare, with a majority occurring in verbal communication settings between clinical staff (Leonard et al., 2004). Therefore, particular attention is needed with respect to designing collaborative technology that supports MDTMs. Information technology can be used to make MDTMs more efficient and collaborative, thereby allowing the medical specialists to make more informed decisions.

7.2   STUDY DESIGN

Our study includes observational fieldwork and cooperative design work spanning two projects over a five-year period starting in Summer 2007. During the first three years the first author, and during the third year also the second author and another researcher, spent an average of 20 h per week at Gastro, performing data collection (approximately 100 h of observing individual surgeons and radiologists, 200 h observing MDTMs among which 40 h have been video recorded, a large number of hours observing and overhearing conversations between surgeons at the Gastro office, 25 formal interviews, a large number of informal interviews, and attending 25 morning meetings at Gastro) in both medical and office environments, as well as sharing the department office and break room. This last opportunity allowed for informal data collection as a side product of ordinary office work by overhearing everyday activities within the office and allowing for impromptu informal discussions. Our orientation to field research follows the approach taken by Hughes et al. (1992), emphasising the description of observable features of the work.

The first period of fieldwork resulted in a joint research project between the medical faculty at the surgical department and HCI researchers from KTH Royal Institute of Technology. The project started in Autumn 2008 aimed at creating simulation and decision support for surgical problems. The first author was the project leader and the second author conducted his Ph.D. work within the project. We adopted a cooperative design methodology (Bødker et al., 2000; Greenbaum & Kyng, 1992) with early user involvement in system and interface design, primarily by using low- and high-tech prototypes. We conducted a number of parallel activities in the project (Frykholm et al., 2010): observations and interviews, project meetings including a larger group of physicians, evaluations of prototypes, workshops and prototyping sessions with a selection of the physicians in the project group, and evaluations at simulated MDTMs. We also included physicians other than those in the project group in the evaluations of prototypes.

At this time ethical approval was needed in order to conduct the detailed data collection needed for the research activities. We needed access to patient information in order to understand what information was needed and to work with realistic data during prototype development, and we needed to video record MDTM sessions to analyse these in detail. However, no patient contact was needed, which made the ethical approval application simpler.

Initially, a series of meetings with all project members, including the group of physicians, was held. These meetings focused on the physicians guiding the HCI researchers in their interpretation of work processes at Gastro, and on the HCI researchers presenting a bird's-eye-view of the work at Gastro. The researchers were invited to collect data for technology development through observing specific situations. Thus, we became involved through an invitation to observe an operation in order to learn what information is available in these situations. This operation, which was a liver resection, was particularly memorable as I (Kristina) remember the awful smell of burned meat that haunted me for several days—not something I was used to.

In addition, early in the project, a number of workshops and demo sessions were conducted to show-case prototypes developed in other projects, including modifications of the prototypes intended to better suit the physicians' needs. The goal was for the physicians to hands-on test the technology and discuss in what ways it could be used in their work. This is in line with Coiera (2007) who suggests that the medical community *"needs to get 'technical' about what we [the medical specialty] mean and about what we want from a design, and we need to work alongside technologists to shape technology, as well as the processes, organizations and cultures within which they will be embedded"*.

Following the initial fieldwork, when project members had cooperatively developed high-level specifications of the intended system, prototyping sessions were conducted to start designing the system interface. Evaluations at varying levels of fidelity were conducted during the prototyping period (Olwal et al., 2011; Sallnäs, 2011).

During 2 three-day sessions at the HCI department, one of the physicians joined three to four researchers in hands-on, cooperative design activities and produced sketches of the system. The prototype was tested and evaluated at two simulated MDTMs one year apart; the first one with five surgeons and two radiologists (Frykholm et al. 2012), and the second one with six surgeons and one radiologist. Real patient data, recorded one to three years earlier, was used in six patient cases that were discussed, three at each of the sessions. One of the surgeons had an active role in the entire design process, while most of the others, but not all, had seen the intended system at different stages of prototyping and evaluation.

In all, the project meetings, fieldwork, prototyping sessions, and evaluations represent a long-term collaboration with Gastro that has helped develop a close relationship between the HCI researchers and the surgeons. The medical specialists could see a potential benefit in how their work process can be improved. Such investment in relationships among project members is critically important.

7.3   STUDY EXPERIENCE

7.3.1   KEY STUDY ENABLERS

The close collaboration with Gastro has been a major success factor. The collaboration started with the first author being invited to do a postdoc in a two-year mediated communication project. This invitation came from the manager at Gastro, a professor of surgery, who during this five-year period became manager of the whole surgical department, and later founded the Innovation Center where both authors are now employed. We met the manager by chance, through a friend of Kristina's who knew two people working with telemedicine development at Gastro. Kristina contacted them, gave them her thesis, and they gave it to the manager. The manager became interested in her HCI background and invited her to meet them and visit one of their MDTMs. This "by chance" contact ended with a postdoctoral position.

The postdoc was the start of a close long-term collaboration and a three-year joint research project between medical specialists from the surgical and radiology departments and the HCI researchers.

It was not just that the manager was the key study enabler, but that this person was visionary, open to new ideas, persuasive, and had a drive for developing new technologies and work processes, which has been crucial for our close and long term collaboration with Gastro. This drive is probably quite unique and not easy to find, but what is important is the influence that the manager had on other clinicians who, in turn, turned into key study enablers themselves. Another important factor was that the manager understood the potential of qualitative research, despite the strong emphasis on quantitative research in the medical community. The manager was very important in providing contacts and giving access to key persons, as well as being a discussant regarding different ideas.

7.3.2   RELATIONSHIPS

The large amount of time that the first author spent in the Gastro office—not only conducting observations and interviews but also just being there—established a close relationship between the HCI researchers and the physicians. The physicians did not only approach the HCI-researchers regarding technical issues (e.g., asking about computer applications) or to tell them stories about things that had happened (e.g., a decision being wrongly documented after an MDTM), but they also initiated discussions on innovative solutions to work related issues (e.g., how to use iPads to access medical records or use video communication to do remote surgical consultations in real time).

The close relationship established through the initial fieldwork made it possible to create a collaborative project including both the physicians and HCI researchers. In this situation, it was important not to "over use" the relationship gained from the initial studies, but to carefully use the physicians as resources in the collaborative project. The time they could spend in the project, for example, in workshops or participating in evaluation sessions, was extremely valuable for us as HCI researchers, but this was a lower priority compared to the time they spent on their clinical work. We had to adapt to their scheduled time in surgery and at outpatient clinics, MDTMs, etc. Meetings with one person were easier to arrange than, for example, workshops including several people. Our close collaboration with one of the surgeons helped us recruit people for workshops.

One problem we encountered was trying to plan the physicians' time on the project. They plan their working schedule three months ahead of time. If we wanted a surgeon to work with us in the project for a couple of days, or even a week, we had to plan that several months ahead. For us, this was not possible because we did not know what activities we would be involved in three months ahead. We were lucky in that one of the head surgeons had time off on two separate occasions when we were ready for prototyping sessions. These two occasions could therefore be planned just a month ahead. Apart from these days, we were able to get the physicians' time every now and then, for them to participate in workshops, etc. The close relationship was probably important in achieving this.

7.3.3   KNOWING THE FIELD

The knowledge of the work at Gastro that the first author gained during the first years, as well as the familiarity with the staff, proved vital in the larger, collaborative project. The first author was able to answer and clarify several questions regarding clinical work from the other HCI researchers.

7.3.4   CONDUCTING COOPERATIVE DESIGN ACTIVITIES

One of our workshops focused on going through the surgeons' work process and the flow of patient information from one activity to another. This workshop did not only give us an insight into their work process and activities, but also enlightened the medical doctors on how they could improve the work process with regard to the lack or loss of information and to prevent breakdowns (Frykholm et al., 2010). One participant commented: *"This is a brilliant way of working with development. [...] Our patient care process makes us light-years ahead. It feels great since we are so far ahead. [...] It's really bracing."*

The close collaboration with one of the surgeons (producing sketches of the system) worked very well. The surgeon was very interested in technology development and had a lot of ideas of what to do. We scheduled two sessions a couple of months apart. The first session focused on getting a first draft of the sketches, which were later evaluated during a workshop with three other surgeons. The second session focused on improving the first sketches based on the evaluation and further development by the HCI researchers.

7.3.5   LACK OF TEST ENVIRONMENTS

The evaluation sessions could be easier to perform if we had access to a test environment within the hospital, including access to medical data. We did have access to seminar rooms at Gastro, and we could use the MDTM room when evaluating the prototype in simulated MDTMs, but it took a large amount of time and effort to set up the studies, especially the simulated MDTMs where we also needed access to the radiology station used to demonstrate images. We did have access to medical data, but we needed to build our own database and use our own computers. Having a test environment at the hospital, where medical data can be accessed and prototypes installed outside the production environment in order to do evaluations, would have been an advantage.

7.3.6   CONDUCTING EVALUATIONS

Our final evaluation workshops—the two where the system was tested in a realistic setting—were most difficult to conduct and took a lot of time to prepare. We needed access to the meeting room in which the MDTMs are held, to a radiologist, and to at least three surgeons. The evaluations also required a large amount of preparation regarding patient cases, logging interaction on the iPads used by the participants during the study session, and planning the study, including making a schedule and designing questions to be discussed after the study session. In the second of the two workshops we also needed to make some installations on the radiology workstation, something that required help from one of the biomedical engineers responsible for the equipment. In the second workshop we also wanted to have one of the surgeons participating over video, but we failed to get this set up. This may have been avoided with a well-prepared test environment.

Whether a personality trait of medical staff in general, or quite specific for the medical specialists we have worked with, they have all along shown a keen interest in our collaborative work and the technical solutions we have presented. For instance, even though they were well aware that the prototypes we tested in simulated MDTMs would never be implemented in the near future, they still made a great effort in making the tests as realistic as possible. In earlier phases of our project, when displaying and testing technical devices of different sorts (Olwal et al., 2011), they could think of several situations in their work where the devices could be used to support a specific work situation. This kind of interest and ingenuity has been inspiring to work with, and has indeed helped to maintain a good relationship with the users over the years.

7.4   CONCLUSIONS

Long-term collaboration, such as we have with Gastro, is a key issue when conducting research in healthcare. The collaboration has been built on a close relationship with the physicians, gained during several years of fieldwork, where a substantial amount of time has been spent on just being in the Gastro office, having informal conversations with the surgeons. The key study enabler—a person with a strong personality, power, and drive regarding development of technology in healthcare—has been very important in our case, but our broader contact with the clinicians has probably been even more important. To establish these contacts we spent hours and hours in their office, something that we believe has been very fruitful. Other success factors include working with them directly on the project, i.e. they were also funded by the project, and sharing our research with them closely. Managing relationships in healthcare is discussed more generally in Volume 2: Chapter 3.

It was difficult for us to make a long-term plan in order to fit our cooperative methods into the physicians' schedules. Instead, we were dependent on them being interested in spending an hour with us every now and then when we needed their input, which they gladly did. We were also lucky to get several days with one of the surgeons to participate in a couple of design workshops.

Finally, a lab environment within the hospital, including access to medical data, where we easily could test prototypes outside the production environment, would have been a benefit. Setting up our own equipment and databases took a lot of time, and some parts were difficult to manage because they interfered with the production environment.

ACKNOWLEDGEMENT

This work was funded by the Celtic project HDViper and the FunkIS project, both funded by VINNOVA. We would like to thank all project colleagues as well as the hospital personnel.

CHAPTER 8

Deploying Healthcare Technology "in the wild:" Experiences from Deploying a Mobile Health Technology for Bipolar Disorder Treatment

Mads Frost and Steven Houben

In this case study, we report on experiences, situations, and lessons learned from working on the MONARCA research project, completed in close collaboration with patients and clinicians from the Affective Disorder Clinic at the University Hospital Copenhagen in Denmark. We discuss aspects of the design, implementation, and evaluation of MONARCA, and summarise some of the key issues and challenges that presented themselves during our work, including:

- Recruiting and motivating mental health patients to participate in healthcare technology research;

- Challenges that occur during data collection, specifically with interviewing mental health patients; and

- Dealing with unintended and surprising consequences in healthcare research.

8.1   RESEARCH FOCUS

There are many important factors to be aware of when doing Human-Computer Interaction (HCI) research in a medical or clinical setting. This chapter describes some of the experiences and lessons learned during the work of deploying the MONARCA Self-Assessment System, a mobile health technology supporting the treatment of bipolar disorder. This work was carried out in collaboration with the Affective Research Unit and the Affective Disorder Clinic at the University Hospital Copenhagen—also known as *Rigshospitalet*—the biggest hospital in Denmark.

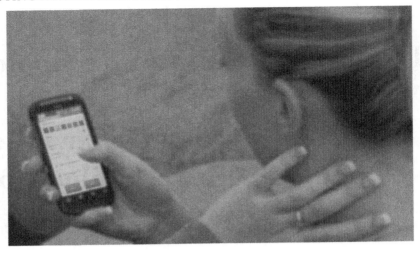

Figure 8.1: A bipolar patient using the MONARCA Android phone application for filling in her self-assessment data by the end of the day.

MONARCA is an abbreviation of MONitoring, treAtment, and pRediCtion of bipolAr Disorder Episodes, hence the central goal of the MONARCA project is to support the treatment of patients suffering from bipolar disorder, a mental illness characterised by recurring episodes of both depression and mania.

The MONARCA system (Bardram et al., 2012) (Frost et al., 2013) consists of two main parts: (i) an Android mobile phone application used exclusively by patients (see Figure 8.1) and (ii) a website used by both patients and clinicians.

By using a personal Smartphone-based application, the patient is provided with a greater awareness of the disease thus allowing him to exercise a much greater degree of self-care and self-treatment. The system allows the patient to self-assess and reviews various health parameters, thereby supporting illness management. For example, patients use the data to keep track of adherence to medication, investigate illness patterns, identify early warning signs for upcoming affective episodes or test potentially beneficial behaviour changes. Additionally, the data collected by the system can be used to predict and prevent the relapse of critical episodes. Through monitoring and feedback, the system helps patients implement effective short-term responses to warning signs and preventative long-term habits. This reduces the need for clinical supervision, treatment, and care, while at the same time empowering the patient in dealing with the disease.

The MONARCA system was designed through a user-centred process, involving both patients and clinicians, who participated in collaborative design workshops, as depicted in Figure 8.2. Three-hour sessions were held every other week over a period of 12 months. These workshops had two main goals: the understanding of how patients were affected by and coped with their illness in daily life, and the identification of the new system's overall goals, detailed system features, and its user interface and graphical design. These requirements evolved gradually and were refined through the hands-on evaluation of paper-based mock-ups and early prototypes of the system (Marcu et al., 2011).

The system first went through a field trial with 12 patients using the system for 12 weeks, to ensure its stability, feasibility, and usability. After this, a randomized clinical trial with 60 patients was undertaken and ran for 2 years where the system's clinical efficacy was assessed. The lessons learned from the first field trial formed the basis for a new iteration of design workshops with patients and clinicians. This resulted in version 2.0 of the system, which was again tested in a field trial with 18 patients for 19 weeks.

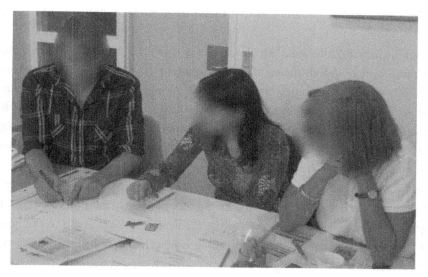

Figure 8.2: A patient, a designer, and a clinician working together on a design activity using prototyping materials.

8.2 STUDY EXPERIENCES

We have summarised some of the key issues that presented themselves during our work. These issues are aligned with the key stages of design, implementation, and evaluation.

First, from the design perspective, we share our experiences of working with mental health patients. We then discuss functional and non-functional challenges, as well as trust and transparency issues from a implementation perspective. Finally, from the evaluation perspective, we describe the unintended effects on the psychological work environment for the clinicians when using the system.

8.2.1   WORKING WITH MENTAL HEALTH PATIENTS

In the MONARCA project, working with mental health patients presented several challenges. We refer here not only the overwhelming experience of witnessing extremely ill patients, suffering from suicidal depression or mania so severe that they needed to be restrained, but also patients whose illness imparted a more subtle effect on their mood and behaviour.

Patients' illnesses could mean that they did not show up, or they could be so influenced by the effects of medication that they were not fully mentally present or even fell asleep. Their depression could mean that they did not have the energy to participate, or they could be so manic that they contributed a host of far-fetched ideas, which needed to be filtered out. As a result, the researchers discovered that it was important to get to know the patients personally, so that when the patients participated in design workshops, any bias that their illness might impart could be better identified and avoided.

For example, one middle-aged female patient was what is referred to in the psychiatric literature as a "rapid cycler," which means that she experiences severe mood swings every 2–3 days, going from highly manic to deeply depressed, and vice versa. The researcher got to know her and her illness so well that when she walked through the door, he could immediately tell what state she was in—just from her appearance. She had an extremely difficult life trying to cope with the disease, but was determined to participate in the design process so that hopefully, others might be spared the "living hell" she felt her life was.

No matter what area of healthcare you are in, at the end of the day, exposure to ill people can be a harsh experience for non-clinical researchers. In mental health, the impact of the illness on the patients' cognitive utilisation and the impact of the medication are not visual to the human eye and thus present additional challenges when performing user-centred design work with patients. It is hard to prepare for, but it is something to be aware of. More perspective on readying the researcher can be found in Volume 2: Chapter 2.

8.2.2   FUNCTIONAL AND NON-FUNCTIONAL CHALLENGES

Deploying healthcare technology "in the wild" brings forth a range of issues when getting the system running. Some are obvious and well known, while other, apparently trivial issues, can be a great hindrance if not addressed. As an HCI researcher, focus is often on the technology aspect of the deployment we are doing in collaboration with patients and hospitals, getting things to work as technically intended. However, there is a big difference between building something that is technically feasible—e.g., getting the functionality in place—and actually having it implemented and running. There are a lot of non-functional aspects that have to be in place for the technology to work, which is key for the success of the project. These non-functional aspects cover everything surrounding the technology, which needs to be in place for it to work as intended. This entails big and small issues, everything from managing the support of the system, the infrastructures, all the way down to the task of creating user guides to hand out to patients and clinicians.

From the MONARCA project there are examples of both functional and non-functional issues, but here we will give a few of the non-functional experiences, as these tend to be those that are most difficult to foresee and handle.

Introducing technology: When introducing patients to a new technological platform such as the Smartphone, ensuring that it will actually be used is dependent not only on whether they know how to use the specific application, but also on whether they know how to use the phone as a whole. The researchers needed to help patients transfer SIM cards from their old phones, and copy their contacts, text messages, images, and other content. A data plan for the patients' 3G connection was needed to enable them to transmit their data from the phone to the hospital's server. If they did not have this, then the researcher helped the patients to contact their provider, set up a data plan, and make the necessary configuration changes on the phone. Besides the setup and the thorough introduction to the phone and our application, it also required preparing user guides and a hotline for technical assistance in the event that patients encountered issues they could not resolve.

Clinical IT unfamiliarity: Another hurdle the researcher encountered during the project was the IT unfamiliarity of the staff at the hospital. For example, the project nurse—the key contact person for the patients and a principal participant in the running of the system—had never dealt with Smartphones before and only knew the basics of how to turn on a computer, check email, and write a Word document. Thus, the researcher spent many hours teaching her not only how to use the system, but about technology in general. Different remote support tools were set up—such as Skype video calls and the ability to remote desktop her computer—so that the researcher was not required to be there in person in order to help her. However, all this entailed communication with and approval from the hospital's IT department, which was often a laborious process.

Being autonomous: Being physically remote from the deployment location presents some challenges when providing help when issues arise. Often, patients would wait to report problems until they came in for an appointment, and the researcher often encountered issues he was not aware of before going to the hospital. Therefore, a portable tool kit for fixing phones and computers was created—everything from extra chargers, network cables, SD cards, cords, covers, software, and even spare phones. This allowed for the handling of most of the issues encountered.

However, due to the use of Smartphones, many of the issues involved the phone itself, rather than the deployed technology. The researcher even experienced a patient presenting a list of different issues she needed help with. Among these items were setting up Skype on the phone so she could talk to her nephew who was attending high school in the U.S. for a year, getting help receiving phone bills as PDFs in her email account, and she even brought her old digital camera along, which she wanted advice on how to operate. This clearly exceeded the boundaries of the deployed technology, but we helped nonetheless.

Scheduling patients: Showing up to visits can be difficult for mental health patients if they are not mentally fit. The researcher's experience with these patients was that they did not show up for nearly 50% of the appointments. As an example, one day five patients were scheduled, starting from nine in the morning until three in the afternoon. The researcher arrived 20 min early to make sure everything was ready for the first patient. And then the waiting started. Out of the 5 patients, 4 of them did not show up and the last one cancelled 13 min prior to the appointment. Thus, the deployment's time planning needs to have leeway to accommodate the impact of patients not showing up to appointments.

In summary, as with any deployment, there are many small things that might seem trivial and not part of the technical solutions, but are extremely important for the success of the technology—especially when dealing with elaborate, pervasive, and multi-user systems. You will do yourself a great favour by considering the possible issues beforehand, to save yourself from later headaches, e.g., try to brainstorm the many possible issues that could go wrong, pilot your project, and seek advice from stakeholders and patients to help foresee potential problems. Fore more guidance on these functional and non-functional challenges see Volume 2: Chapter 5.

8.2.3 TRUST AND TRANSPARENCY

The attribution of trust indicates a positive belief about the perceived reliability of, dependability of, and confidence in a person, object, or process. Trust is especially important in healthcare, as we are dealing with highly personal and potentially life critical information.

In MONARCA, a voice analysis feature was implemented, where the application would record the first two minutes of a patient's phone call, encrypt it, analyse it in terms of e.g., loudness of speech, frequencies, length of talk, and a range of other features—thus, analysing not what was said but how it was said. When the analysis was completed, the system would delete the recording and save the results in the database. The hypothesis is that it is possible to assess the patient's mood from these voice features.

However, one day one of the patients called the hotline, stating that he had uninstalled the application. He explained that he was using the phone and was about to listen to music. He plugged in the earphones and suddenly heard his father talking. He got confused and started answering "hello, hello?!?" but his father just kept on talking. Then he heard his own voice replying to his father, and realised that it was a recording of a previous phone call conversation. He examined the SD-card on the phone, and found two unencrypted phone call recordings, even though the app had gone through extensive testing before release. When it was discovered, the feature was immediately removed, and an update was released, and all patients' phones were checked—fortunately no one else experienced the same issue. But it led to an interesting conversation with the patient on how he was glad that he was neutral when this happened, as he at times suffered from paranoia, and this could really have pushed him off balance. After this event, and curious about what we actually had access to on his phone, he checked the *Google Play* market. He knew which bits of information we were monitoring from all the information he had received from us, but when going through the market, it said that the application had access to a lot more than what we expressed we gathered. For instance, it took some time to explain that even though it said the application had access to his text messages, it simply counted the number of messages sent and received, and did not access the content of the messages. As he explained, it was not that he did not trust the researchers and the application, but that what was going on "under the hood" was not transparent enough. He reinstalled the app after the update was issued, and finished the trial without any hesitation.

Building a trustworthy relationship with participants helps ensure their commitment and willingness to provide intimate personal data, and is strengthened by transparency in both systems and actions. This depicts a need for transparency in the technology issued, which can be a complicated matter when we are dealing with platforms and infrastructures we do not fully control.

8.2.4   UNINTENDED EFFECTS

When building and evaluating interventions in healthcare systems, the key focus is on the effect and the safety of the patients—but the clinicians are users of the system as well. In the user-centred design process of the MONARCA system, we spent a considerable amount of time and effort establishing how the system would be integrated into the treatment process at the hospital, and how the clinicians should act according to the data from the patients. During the trials there was a change from a reactive to a proactive treatment approach, because clinicians now had access to data that they did not have access to before. The clinicians who were monitoring the patients on a daily basis felt it is a big responsibility to assess which patients needed to be contacted to make sure everything was going well. Difficult questions would arise when they could see a patient's data starting to change. When was the change big enough to perform an early intervention, and when should they wait and follow-up the day after? There were predefined rules for when contact should be made, but the clinicians still sometimes worried about whether they had made the right decision. This was especially the case for clinicians covering for others while they were sick or on holiday, and were not involved in the regular treatment of the specific patient, and thus did not know the impact of the changes to the same extent as the patient's regular clinician.

Another example was when the system had no connection to a patient's phone for several days. Given there had been no connection, the system could not know what caused this—it could be the patient had forgotten to turn on the phone, it had run out of power, they accidently uninstalled the app, the internet connection was turned off, or that the phone had been broken or stolen, but it could also be that the patient was ill and did not want to turn on the phone or simply could not. In any case, the clinician did not know the cause of this lack of data, and the effect of being the one responsible for the patients was troublesome for the clinicians. The easy solution was to call the patient and ask what caused this, but if there were no answer, questions arose on how to handle this "data blindness." Should the clinicians call the relatives of the patient, risking giving them a scare when everything was fine? And if this did not succeed, should they go to the patient's home to ensure the patient was doing okay? These issues were especially troublesome on Fridays, as the clinicians would not log into the system again until Monday morning. Some clinicians stated that they could spend all weekend thinking about these patients, and some even logged in over the weekend, just to keep track of how the patients progressed.

This insight, or more importantly the lack of insight, into how the patients were doing was an additional stress factor for the clinicians when using the system. The work practices were addressed to handle this additional mental load. Even though the effects of systems for users other than the actual patients are not the key focus for the work with interventions in healthcare, these are extremely important to include and consider in a design process, to avoid unnecessary problems and work loads—mental or physical.

8.3   CONCLUSIONS

Clinical research in collaboration with hospitals or other medical partners provides HCI researchers with interesting opportunities but also poses difficult challenges related to this domain. In this case study, we presented a few of these challenges that we encountered during the fieldwork for the MONARCA project.

We reported on experiences with working with mental health patients in design situations, the functional and non-functional challenges that need to be addressed when deploying systems in order to ease the deployment, the importance of focus on trust and transparency of such systems in order to make the patients feel safe, and finally also keeping focus on the other users in these systems and the effect that interventions can have on their work practice.

ACKNOWLEDGEMENT

We thank all the patients, clinicians, and researchers we have had the pleasure of working with in the project. The MONARCA project is funded as a EU FP7 STREP project—see http://monarca-project.eu/.

CHAPTER 9

Designing Technology for Extremely Vulnerable Adults: The Important Role of Staff in Design and Ethics

Anja Thieme, Paula Johnson, Jayne Wallace, Patrick Olivier, and
Thomas D. Meyer

We report on our on-going research in designing interactive technology for female patients in the forensic services of a U.K. hospital. These women represent a very vulnerable group due to the severity of their mental health problems, extremely challenging behaviours, and their motivational difficulties in engaging in therapeutic treatment. This case study details the approaches we have taken in addressing the challenges faced whilst planning this research, specifically:

- The importance of close collaboration with hospital staff in gaining an in-depth understanding of specific design contexts;

- Collaboration can be crucial for addressing related ethical demands for the design of the technology, as well as for identifying appropriate evaluation methods; and

- Issues specific to research involving sensitive patient groups in intense healthcare settings.

9.1   RESEARCH FOCUS

This research focuses on the design and evaluation of a set of interactive artefacts (the *Spheres of Wellbeing*) that are specifically developed for a group of six women in secure services of a U.K. hospital, to support them in the learning and practice of vital therapeutic skills. The women commonly suffer from a dual diagnosis of a Learning Disability (LD) and Borderline Personality Disorder (BPD). The women's LD is usually mild to moderate, which causes them some difficulties in understanding, learning, and problem solving, limits their attention span, and impacts on their interactions and communications with other people (Chilvers et al., 2011; Robertson, 2011).

BPD is mainly characterised by severe difficulties in regulating, interpreting, or tolerating emotions. As a result, the women tend to be very sensitive and responsive to emotional cues and lack the ability to self-sooth physiological arousal induced through strong emotions (Linehan,

1993). In attempting to cope for instance with intense emotional pain, they often engage in behaviours which promise distraction or immediate relief, such as impulsive behaviours, inappropriate anger outbursts and acts of self-harm (Yen et al., 2002). They also show a variety of cognitive disturbances (e.g., they overvalue the idea of being bad, or believe that they do not deserve anything nice) and have profound difficulties in forming and maintaining stable social relationships (Lieb et al., 2004; Linehan, 1993).

9.1.1 INITIATION OF THIS RESEARCH

Driven by a general research need to improve the lives of people with poor health and disability, this project came about through a hospital visit by one of the researchers, who was shown around the secure services and introduced to the particularly challenging and severe condition of the women. Ideas for the research were then developed through further visits by members of the research team to the hospital, which enabled us to spend time with staff nurses and therapists working directly with the women and to talk to members of the Research and Development (R&D) team. For more information on how to establish and maintain relationships with hospital staff see Volume 2: Chapter 3.

9.1.2 CLOSE COLLABORATION WITH HOSPITAL STAFF

During brainstorming activities, clinicians shared with us materials and contents they use in therapy. We were able to present them with examples of previous research projects that were characteristic of our person-focused design approach, and that would introduce them to commonly applied methods in HCI (e.g., probes and participatory design). Through this process, hospital staff could gain a better understanding of the rich opportunities offered by digital designs. It was also crucial for us to develop an understanding of the complex psychiatric condition of the women, recommended treatment approaches, the safety regulations of the secure services, and related issues regarding research governance and ethics.

A mutual understanding of each other's practices was further facilitated by the fortunate circumstance that some of the hospital staff were both clinically experienced and research-oriented. The R&D manager is a trained Cognitive Behavioural Therapist who had been working in the women's services for more than 15 years, and one of the staff nurses was interested in supporting the research as part of her Master's degree. The basic design and functionality of the *Spheres* were established in our meetings with hospital staff and were informed by the literature about the mental health condition of the women and their treatment program.

9.2   THE SPHERES OF WELLBEING

9.2.1   DESIGN CONCEPT AND RATIONALE

The *Spheres of Wellbeing* is a set of three artefacts designed to support the women in learning and practicing the vital skills of their specialised treatment: Dialectical Behavioural Therapy (Linehan, 1993). These include mindful awareness, the tolerance of emotional distress, and the promotion of a strong sense of self.

The *Mindfulness Sphere* (see Figure 9.1) is a ball-shaped artefact that assesses and reflects a person's heart rate through colourful lights. As such, the ball can invite a new, experiential way of bringing awareness to one's body and—as a form of biofeedback—offers the opportunity to regulate an aspect of one's self.

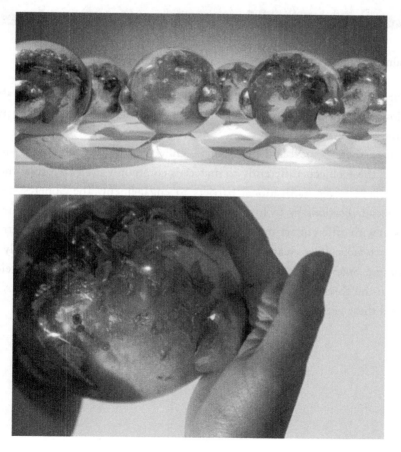

Figure 9.1: The six personalised Mindfulness Spheres of the women (top), and a close up of one of the Spheres (bottom).

The *Calming Sphere* (see Figure 9.2) is a non-digital bead bracelet that the women can hold on to at times of emotional distress.

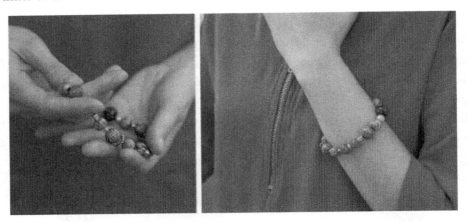

Figure 9.2: A Calming Sphere bracelet with beads made by each of the women.

The *Identity Sphere* (see Figure 9.3) gently invites the women to engage with short personalised videos, allowing them to explore and reconnect to meaningful aspects of their self (for more details, see Thieme et al., 2012; 2013).

A focus on aesthetic appeal and physicality—enlivened by the technology—may lead the women to perceive these objects differently to materials commonly used in formal therapy, which can reduce stigma and lower motivational barriers to engagement. The Spheres' design further leaves space for personalisations by each woman. In creative activities with one of the researchers, the women worked with different art and craft materials for the creation of visually attractive pieces for their Spheres artefacts. They created beautiful little plastic images that are visibly encased inside their *Mindfulness Sphere*, made their own clay beads for the *Calming Sphere* bracelet, and were actively involved in the co-creation of the personalised videos of their *Identity Sphere*. The women very much enjoyed these activities and were proud of their creations.

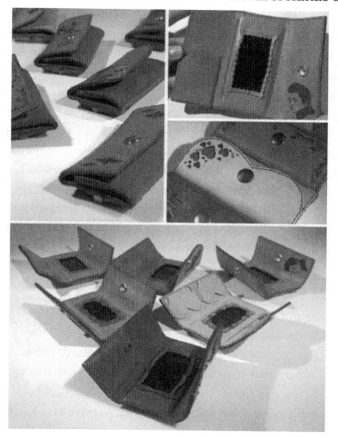

Figure 9.3: The personalised Identity Spheres of the women: Purse-like artefacts that display personally meaningful videos on the screen inside, triggered by QR codes.

9.2.2   STAFF INPUT AND INFORMAL EVALUATIONS

The designs benefited from discussions with clinicians and R&D staff who primarily raised concerns about the safety of the objects (e.g., risks of self-harm through access to batteries or sharp metal pieces) and the materials for the co-creative activities. To this end, tear proof, robust materials have been used in the designs to safely encase the technology, such as resin for the Mindfulness Sphere or leather for the Identity Sphere, and we were briefed about the safety procedures in place (e.g., individual risk assessments of each woman, supervision of all research activities by staff).

Our conversations also included debates about whether the Spheres are "medical devices," defined by the National Health Service (NHS) as *"any instrument, apparatus, appliance, material or healthcare product, excluding drugs, used for a patient or client for the purposes of diagnosis, prevention, monitoring, treatment or alleviation of disease*"[2] (p. 36). Although the Spheres incorporate technology to assess the women's heart rate, it is not intended to monitor their pulse for any medical purposes. Instead the Sphere responds dynamically to the women to allow for interesting, stimulating experiences when engaging in therapeutic exercises. As such, it acts more like a teaching aid than a medical device and thus our ethics procedures and our study plans reflected this (this point is expanded in this book's companion volume on guidance).

Overall, staff were enthusiastic about the designs, and assessed them to be appropriate for use in the secure services and as an addition to the women's treatment. They appreciated the physicality and visual presence of the objects, particularly for women with LD, providing them with something to hold on to and that presents a visual reminder of their therapy. They valued that the women actively contributed to their designs, and predicted that interactions with the objects are likely to be intriguing to them. The following outlines our decision making process in the design of an evaluative study of the Spheres with the women.

9.3   STUDY DESIGN AND ETHICS

Potential participants of this research were identified by their clinical care team, following a list of specific inclusion and exclusion criteria. Due to the women's LD, we specified that the women needed to be able to give consent (as assessed by their care team) and have sufficient ability to express themselves to ensure that they understood the project and also to minimize additional ethical concerns.

Since the women represent a very vulnerable group, we were asked, in the meeting with our Research Ethics Committee (REC), how we planned to ensure that the women did not feel pressured into taking part. The R&D manager of the hospital, who also attended the meeting, assured the REC that the hospital follows a very person-centred approach and that the women are generally very assertive and would not take part unless they really wanted to. Such ethically important client group specific information often needs to be worked out locally. For more information on research governance and ethics see Volume 2: Chapter 1.

As part of the process of seeking consent, the women were first carefully introduced to the project. To this end, we showed them examples of the Spheres as well as of craft materials, and explained the purpose of the creative activities. The women were then provided with an information sheet, written in easily accessible language and supported by pictorial prompts, which we talked through together. Following best practice in the process of seeking consent, the women were given sufficient time (in this case up to one week) to carefully reflect on and discuss their potential participation with others, before written consent was sought from those who volunteered.

---

[2] NHS Bolton, Medical Devices & Equipment Management Policy, 2008. Last retrieved 19.12.2012, http://www.bolton.nhs.uk/Library/policies/RM032.pdf

9.3.1   SAFETY, HEALTH, AND WELLBEING OF ALL INVOLVED

The creative sessions took place on the women's ward to protect the health and wellbeing of all involved: this environment was familiar to the women, so it could reduce any anxieties they may have had, and it provided the advantage that staff support was available at all times (e.g., if the women became emotionally distressed). The research activities were at all times accompanied by at least one regular member of staff, which significantly reduced most risks but created organisational and financial demands. Both staff and the researcher further had to wear an alarm system whenever they were on the ward, for use in an emergency. In addition, the researcher also attended "breakaway training," where she was taught how to maintain a safe distance from the women or how to block an attack, and had to adhere to the safety procedures in place (e.g., the counting in and out of all materials brought onto the ward). Since interactions with particularly challenging and sensitive client groups—like the women in this project—can affect the emotional wellbeing of the researcher, access to counselling support should be considered.

To avoid upsetting the women, the researcher was briefed by staff about certain sensitive topics that should be avoided in conversations with individual women (e.g., disrupted family relations) and about specific behavioural risks (e.g., a woman's tendency to pull hair). However, at no time did the researcher have access to the forensic histories of the women, as they were not essential for the conduct of this research. Accessing this data would require the women to first give their consent, which could be challenging, as the women tend to be embarrassed about their personal history and are often unwilling to let others know about it, with the risk that they may reject participation entirely. These insights and our approach to appropriately address the ethical issues of this research are closely informed by our collaboration with hospital staff who shared with us their in-depth experiences in conducting research with the women.

9.3.2   EVALUATION METHODOLOGY

Once all Sphere artefacts were finalised, we sat with each woman individually to present her with her set of Spheres, and to encourage explorations of each object. In demonstrating their different functionalities, we worked towards showing potential uses of the objects as a means for therapeutic skills practice. The introductory session also allowed us to manage certain expectations that the women might have of the artefacts (e.g., we reminded them that any technology can break).

To gain a holistic understanding of the women's perceptions and experience of their Spheres, mixed qualitative and quantitative data was collected over a period of four weeks, and a three-month follow-up evaluation was planned. The data set included any materials from the creative sessions, log file data of the women's interactions with the two digital Spheres (i.e., time and frequency of use), documented staff observations, and audio-recorded interviews with the women and staff. For more information on data collection and evaluation methods see Volume 2: Chapter 4.

9.3.3 THE VITAL ROLE OF STAFF SUPPORT

Staff nurses and support workers on the unit played a vital role in modelling pro-social behaviour and assisting the women in attending to their treatment targets, and thus may also be crucial in the process of empowering the women to engage with the Spheres. Staff support in the deployment and evaluation of the Spheres could be viewed as a confounding factor when evaluating the Spheres' effectiveness, as their close involvement in the delivery may conflict with the aims of the research and scientific standards of objectivity. However, their involvement was crucial for various reasons: (i) staff are in continuous contact with the women (unlike the researcher), which can facilitate less intrusive observations of their interactions with the Spheres; (ii) due to their extensive experience of working with the women, staff may also be better at recognising new, unusual, or noteworthy behaviours of the women; and (iii) staff will have to look after the objects (e.g., re-charge them) and can encourage their use.

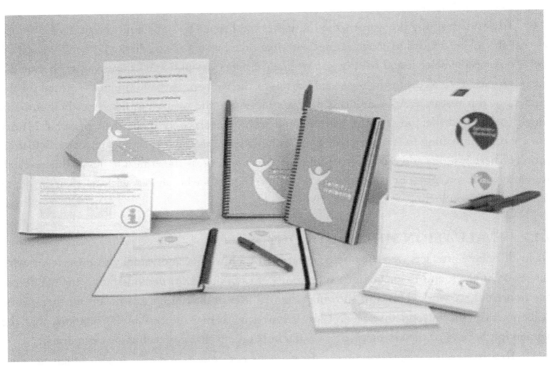

Figure 9.4: *Journals* and *event cards* for the recording of staff observations of the women's engagements with their Spheres of Wellbeing objects. Event cards come in the size of a postcard that, once completed, are placed in a locked post-box in the staff office.

To this end, we provided staff on the unit with *journals* for weekly records of their narrative observations of the women's engagements with the Spheres, and *event cards* to record observations *in situ* (see Figure 9.4). Staff were given explicit instructions and examples of events to carefully provide guidance for less research-experienced staff, and to help reduce observer biases. These materials were chosen because they offer more flexibility, given the burdens of a hectic ward, particularly when compared to other forms of experience sampling (e.g., interval or signal sampling). Participating staff were given additional wage payments for their extra time spent in supporting the research.

9.3.4 GAINING ETHICAL APPROVAL

The study design was approved by the NHS REC and the Research Committee of the Hospital Trust. Recruitment to the research commenced in January 2013. For this to happen, we submitted a detailed protocol of the research, including two independent external reviews, completed the required online ethics forms, provided all study-related documents (e.g., information sheets), as well as evidence of funding, sponsorship, insurance, and a financial agreement contract. In order for non-clinical HCI researchers to gain access to the unit, we each had to apply for a Research Passport, requiring a criminal records check (CRB), Occupational Health clearance, and with this research being an NIHR portfolio study,[3] a certificate of Good Clinical Practice (GCP) training.

To obtain all these necessary documents was a complex and lengthy process that took us approximately 12 months to complete, alongside the conduct of other additional research activities. Partly this is due to the required detail—a useful process of clarifying proposed research activities and how specific risks would be addressed—and partly due to extended waiting periods for certain approvals to come through.

9.4 CONCLUSIONS

Throughout the planning of this research, our close collaboration with hospital staff has been fundamental to our understanding of this sensitive design context. Staff introduced us to the complex mental health condition of the women, their therapy program as well as the safety and ethical requirements of the secure services. They made valuable contributions to informal iterations of early design ideations and evaluations of the Spheres prototypes. For the design of the Spheres and our evaluative study, we tried to balance the various safety, ethical, and organisational requirements of the clinical context—to safeguard the women and to fit into the intense care environment—with our more open-ended ideas and research methods (i.e., creative sessions for the personalisation of pre-defined objects).

[3] http://www.crncc.nihr.ac.uk/about_us/processes/portfolio

ACKNOWLEDGEMENT

This work is supported by Microsoft Research through its Ph.D. Scholarship Programme and the RCUK Digital Economy Hub on Social Inclusion through the Digital Economy (SiDE). We thank all staff at Calderstones for their great support of this research.

CHAPTER 10

The Challenges of Interviewing Older People in Their Own Homes: Reflections and Suggestions from the Field

Ross Thomson, Jennifer L. Martin, and Sarah Sharples

This case study describes some of the challenges encountered during a qualitative, interview-based study concerned with the experience of older people using medical devices in their home. It provides suggestions and ideas for other researchers on how they may navigate similar research areas, including:

- Issues around recruitment of patients for healthcare technology studies;

- Specific issues and opportunities that arise from conducting research in the home environment;

- Challenges related to interviewing older adults; and

- Dealing with emotions when conducting studies directly with patients.

10.1 RESEARCH FOCUS

This case study is based on research we conducted investigating home use medical devices and older people. As a result of an aging population and drive towards a more community-based healthcare system, an increasing number of older people are likely to experience medical technologies in their homes. Much of the human factors literature to date has focused on specific medical technologies in relation to safety and usability. The aim of our study was to collect and analyse qualitative data in an attempt to learn how medical devices are integrated into the lives of older people and understand the psychological and social impact of this process. The qualitative method chosen was a thematic analysis, as proposed by Braun and Clarke (2006), which utilises transcripts of in-depth semi-structured interviews to identify, analyse, and report patterns (themes) within data.

The plan was to conduct and record interviews with older people (65 year plus) from the local area who were currently medical device users, in a place that was convenient for them. In reality most interviews occurred in the participants' own homes.

10.2   RECRUITMENT: NEGOTIATION AND NETWORKS

Recruitment of participants for any study can be challenging and gaining access to potentially vulnerable groups (for example, older people) can be particularly difficult.

Following ethical clearance from the University of Nottingham, I initially started recruitment by advertising our study with posters placed in the university and in targeted locations where I considered it likely that they would be seen by older people, such as Post Offices, shops, and churches. I also placed an advertisement in the local press. While these approaches were not entirely fruitless, the uptake was disappointingly low.

I then tried a different approach, which involved approaching patient and older people's groups. This required a great deal of negotiation with gatekeepers to access these groups (see Volume 2: Chapter 3) . While gatekeepers provide an important function within these groups as a way of protecting some of the more vulnerable members from unsolicited contact, some of the responses we received about our study were less positive than I expected. For example, the organisers of some local groups I contacted replied that they thought that their members would not be interested and that they saw little point in putting it to their membership.

The national charity groups that we approached required a study proposal to be reviewed by their senior management. In this instance, although we were denied the opportunity to address potential participants face to face, we were told that they would distribute details via their newsletter. Again, I received no responses and was becoming frustrated with the whole recruitment process. I could not understand people's reluctance to get involved (either by promoting the study or becoming a participant) given the relatively uncomplicated nature of taking part and that we were offering a reasonable "inconvenience allowance" of £10 shopping vouchers.

Gaining access to older people can be difficult at the best of times but I believe that because I was interested in health related issues the recruitment process was made inherently more difficult. Whether this was because older people with health issues felt increasingly vulnerable and wary is not clear but it certainly added a layer of complexity as I had to liaise with people whose role was to protect this particular group of individuals. I then began to wonder if there was anything I could do to make *myself* more acceptable to potential participants? In the U.K., working with older people in an official position requires a Criminal Records Bureau (CRB) check to help protect the vulnerable. In a bid to ease any concerns the individuals or groups may have had, I applied for a CRB check through the university. While I was never asked to produce my CRB documentation, I did mention my CRB clearance whenever possible as I felt I needed to do as much as I could to alleviate people's concerns and increase my own credibility with people involved with older people.

The recruitment method that proved the most fruitful was snowball sampling (getting participants to recommend/introduce other participants), which is an often used "tactic" to reach "hidden" or marginalised populations (Noy, 2008). The wife of one participant in our study was an active member of the community and other people contacted us to participate in the study as a result of her recommendation. It is this kind of opportunity that highlights the importance of networking and making a good impression on people to help with the challenges recruitment brings.

What I really learned from this experience is to persevere, be prepared to negotiate with gatekeepers, and use different types of sampling methods to reach potential participants.

10.3   PARTICIPANT AND INTERVIEWER SAFETY

A different kind of risk assessment is required with fieldwork of this type. Not only do participants need to feel safe but the safety of the interviewer also needs to be taken into consideration.

For older people, inviting strangers into your house can be a source of anxiety, especially if you feel vulnerable or live on your own. In order for the participant to feel safe in this situation, all interviewees were offered the option of having a chaperone present during the interview. However, none felt they needed this provision. Most of the participants in our study lived with a partner or spouse who was present at the time, which itself gave rise to issues which will be discussed below.

Having previously worked in a community healthcare role, I was particularly aware of how important it was to consider the safety of the interviewer when visiting people in their own homes. These considerations should include travelling to and from the interview as well as entering an unfamiliar environment (see Volume 2: Chapter 2 for a wider discussion of safety concerns).

I mainly used public transport so all trips were planned well in advance and I carried timetables and maps with me. In order to avoid becoming a target for theft while travelling, objects such as laptops and mobile phones were kept out of sight and a lone working procedure was adopted where someone would know where I was going and would receive a phone call after the interview to confirm that all was well.

The safety of the interviewer within the participant's home also requires consideration. For example, one participant in our study owned a large dog. I have to admit that I do get nervous around dogs that I do not know, and a bad experience in my previous job where I was growled at for an hour while I was trying to help its owner has done little to help my confidence. Seeing the participant's dog made me very nervous and I just wanted to leave. Knowing I would be unable to concentrate and give the interview my full attention, I asked if the dog could be kept in another room while the interview took place. This had to be negotiated with sensitivity, as the dog was a treasured member of the household.

This example emphasises the importance of a continual risk assessment process when conducting lone research in the field.

10.4   HEALTHCARE INTERVIEWING

The research interview has been defined as a "professional conversation" in that it is not a "conversation between equal partners" as the aim is to elicit information from the participant (Kvale, 1996). However, it has been suggested that this method of interviewing perpetuates the disempowerment of vulnerable groups (such as older people) and that an equal or dialogical approach should be taken (Russell, 1999), which is what I did my best to achieve.

The interviews in our study certainly benefited from this second approach in terms of rapport building and breaking down barriers between interviewer and interviewee in an attempt to get participants to speak openly. I found it is better to approach the interview as more of a social encounter. While a brief telephone call or email may have confirmed that the participant met the inclusion criteria for the study, it is only after knocking on the door and being invited in that you meet each other for the first time and it is this period that will set the tone of the interview. After usually being offered a drink, I would engage in some small talk ("looks like it's going to rain again!" or "is that a picture of your grandchildren?") to put the participant and myself at ease before going through paperwork, gaining consent, and starting the interview proper. After the interview had ended, I continued with the small talk while packing away equipment and sorting out paperwork. This seemed a more natural way to finish the visit, rather that briskly gathering things together and rushing off, which could leave the participant feeling unhappy or disappointed with the whole encounter.

It is worth noting that in the field of healthcare, older people are more likely to be prone to gratitude and satisfaction bias, particularly in publicly funded services such as the National Health Service (NHS). It has been shown that older people can be reluctant to criticise, will express greater levels of satisfaction with regards to healthcare, and have a tendency to gloss over any negative concerns they have about services and treatments (Calnan et al., 2003; Øvretveit, 1992). It was felt that in our study this was definitely the case as many of the participants reported that they had participated out of a sense of "gratitude" and wanting to give something back. In this respect we found it increasingly important to point out that we were not part of the NHS and emphasised that they should speak freely as anonymity and confidentiality would mean that any criticisms would not reflect on them. Whether we were successful in this is unclear. While I could have asked negative questions about the devices ("what don't you like about your device?") or given examples of what other people had said about their devices, I felt that this would have been leading the participant. I wanted to understand the issues that were important to the participants and which originated from them.

10.5   CONSIDERATIONS IN USING THE HOME ENVIRONMENT

Undertaking qualitative research in people's own homes presents its own challenges. In direct contrast to the controlled environments of laboratories, being invited into another person's personal and private space relinquishes much of that control to the participant and the influences of outside sources. In our study, all but two interviews were carried out in participant homes.

As mentioned previously, having the partner/spouse present in the room during the interview produced its own challenges. The partners we encountered showed more than a passing interest in the study and were keen to listen in on the interview. It would have been awkward to have to exclude a person from a room in their own house and, if the participant agreed, then the partner stayed in the room while the interview took place. These partners, however, were not silent observers and in fact contributed what turned out to be rich data to the study. It was clear that it was not just the patients (as users of medical technology in the home) that were interacting with these devices but the partners were also affected. It quickly became apparent that we needed to also gain consent from the partners in order to use the data. It was acknowledged however that interviewing the user and partner together might have resulted in a less open and frank discussion.

Carrying out research in the home does have advantages, however. The participants in this study were very keen to show me their medical devices (one participant even brought her blood pressure monitor to the university with her for the interview), where they were kept, and how they were used. As I was interested in the integration of these devices into the lives of participants, these "in the field" revelations were instrumental in stimulating further questions and prompts to the semi-structured interviews.

The important thing to remember when conducting research in the home environment is the need for adaptability. While fieldwork in participants' homes is unpredictable and a lot of the time you will be led by the situation, it may also present opportunities not found in other environments that may be of benefit to the study.

10.6   EMOTIONAL CHALLENGES

Talking about medical related topics and interviewing participants with medical conditions can invariably stir emotions in both the participant and the interviewer that may affect the interview.

I found that I needed to be sensitive to the participants' emotional state and on occasion had to modify the order in which questions were asked. For example, one gentleman with a respiratory condition became tearful when explaining how his health was responsible for the loss of long held friendships and the reason he was unable to keep his pets. As a result, I shifted the focus of the questions from negative to more positive aspects of what the medical device had enabled him to do. The negative aspects were revisited later in the interview and framed in different ways. While it would be unethical to offer advice to participants who were upset, I felt it was appropriate to provide all participants with the contact details of support organisations.

Being invited into the homes of people with medical conditions can also be an emotional experience for the interviewer. All the interviewees talked about loss, and death was a frequent topic raised by participants. I had previously worked with older people in the healthcare setting and I felt this experience was extremely valuable in engaging with these emotions. I also allowed myself time to reflect on the emotional issues that arose in each interview and I had the opportunity to debrief matters with a supervisor.

Healthcare as an emotive subject is one that can affect both the participant and the interviewer (see Volume 2: Chapter 2 for a broader discussion of emotion in fieldwork for healthcare). I found that spending a little time thinking and preparing for these issues helped make a potentially difficult or painful encounter more comfortable.

10.7   CONCLUSION

Fieldwork, especially when carried out in people's homes, presents many challenges not normally encountered with lab-based studies. Recruitment of older people and being invited into participants' lives as part of the research involves the transfer of control to a large extent to other people. While meticulous planning is required in any type of study, I found that being flexible enough to react to changing circumstances, as and when they occurred, was the key to the successful completion of this study. I hope that my reflections and the learning points covered here will help other researchers to deal with some of the difficulties that can be encountered when conducting research in the home environment.

ACKNOWLEDGEMENT

The authors gratefully thank the interviewees for participating in the research. The authors also wish to acknowledge support from the EPSRC through the MATCH programme (EP/F063822/1). The views expressed are those of the authors alone.

CHAPTER 11

Studying Patients' Interactions with Home Haemodialysis Technology: The Ideal and The Practical

Atish Rajkomar, Ann Blandford, and Astrid Mayer

In this case study, we reflect on the methods we used to investigate how renal patients and carers interact with home haemodialysis technology. The goal of our study was to understand the interaction issues that patients and carers face and how technology design could be improved for use in the home. Specifically, this chapter covers:

- Being open to changes in research approaches to suit the healthcare setting;

- Limitations on the methods that can be used with sick patients and what they can contribute during data collection; and

- Interview techniques that can be used to elicit information about home technologies.

11.1 RESEARCH FOCUS

As healthcare shifts to the home environment, patients and carers take responsibility for treatment and become the main users of healthcare technology. Taking home haemodialysis as an example, our research investigates how patients and carers interact with healthcare technology in the home. Home haemodialysis is a treatment for patients suffering from kidney failure. During treatment, a patient's blood gets cleaned as it flows into a special filter, which is connected to a machine. In our study, we focused on understanding the contexts in which renal patients and carers interact with home haemodialysis technology, the interaction issues they face, and how they cope with these issues. These insights can help inform the design of safe and patient-friendly home healthcare technology.

11.2   STUDY DESIGN

11.2.1   GAINING ACCESS TO THE FIELD

Initially, we started the processes for getting the different permissions required to study the use of medical devices in three settings: the use of home haemodialysis machines by renal patients of one hospital; the use of ambulatory infusion pumps by palliative care nurses of another hospital in patient's homes; and the use of ambulatory infusion pumps by nurses of a hospice. These permissions include National Health Service (NHS) ethics approval and hospital-specific Research & Development (R&D) approval. During the process of getting ethics approval, the opportunity to study infusion pump use by palliative care nurses in homes phased out, seemingly due to organisational changes.

It took six months to get all the permissions to start the first home haemodialysis study and the study of infusion pump use in the hospice. Attempts were made to gain access to home patients through non-NHS routes also, firstly by contacting some home healthcare providers and secondly by contacting some organisations that represent patients. The first route was unsuccessful, while the second route led to one participant being recruited, through an open letter that was posted on the website of the National Kidney Federation.

11.2.2   PARTICIPANT RECRUITMENT

Participants were recruited for the first home haemodialysis study through the home nurse. The home nurse informed the hospital's home patients who she considered could be potential participants of the study, and then arranged for us to contact interested patients. We then arranged for home visits. During the first home visit to each patient, a participant information sheet was given to the patient, and the purpose of the study was explained to them, before recording their consent on a consent form. The participant information sheet and consent form were both approved by the hospital's R&D office, and different versions had to be produced for staff members, patients, and carers.

In parallel with the home haemodialysis study, a study of nurses' use of infusion pumps in the hospice was started. However, due to uncertainties to do with the continuation of the use of the pumps and with anticipated organisational changes, that study was abandoned. In a sense, our project to study medical device use in the home was eventually successful because we started with three possibilities: only the home haemodialysis study materialised. This highlights the importance of considering several possibilities when planning such studies.

11.2.3   DATA GATHERING APPROACH

Our approach was to work with patients and carers as co-researchers in understanding and critiquing the design of the technology that they use (Blandford et al., 2009). To do this, we initially planned to gather data on how patients and carers interact with dialysis technology mainly by loaning them handheld video recorders to keep diaries and capture minor incidents. This data would be supplemented with observations, interviews, analyses of device behaviour through bench tests, institutional data on actual incidents, and consultation of system/device manuals. The rationale for requesting patients and carers to keep diaries was that it could be a potentially effective solution to the privacy issue of gathering data in the home setting. From the outset, this was an exploratory approach, which would be adapted based on how well it worked in practice. We conducted a preliminary study with five patients and their carers. The preliminary study was meant to inform subsequent studies on which data gathering techniques work well, and proved to be crucial for the success of our project.

11.3   STUDY EXPERIENCE

11.3.1   DIARIES NOT A VIABLE APPROACH

In the preliminary study, three participants agreed to keep handheld video recorders to capture incidents with the technology. However, only one of them made a recording, and of only one interaction. One participant who self-cares mentioned that, when an incident happened, it was not practical for him to hold the recorder in one hand and try to fix the problem with the other hand (we provided them with stands, but this still requires them to carefully adjust the position and angle of the camera). Another participant, who is a carer, mentioned that when an incident happens, his reflex is to fix the problem as soon as possible, and not to record it. The two other participants, who did not keep video recorders, were not willing to keep pen and paper diaries either, as they already had to maintain dialysis charts. They occasionally noted down incidents on these charts, and allowed me to consult them.

The participants understandably did not have the time, energy, or enthusiasm to invest even more time in their dialysis activity. The dialysis treatment setup, the treatment itself, the overall management of the treatment (including, for example, managing and ordering medical supplies), and related hospital appointments, consume so much of the time of patients and carers that some struggle to make any free time to do other activities in their personal lives. Also, there are many steps involved in the preparation and conduct of the treatment, and it is not uncommon for them to forget to do one or two things. Additionally, the dialysis treatment has side effects (such as decreasing the blood pressure of the patient), which very often make patients feel lethargic or nauseous or headachy during and after the treatment. Alarms during the treatment are frequent, and can be a very stressful experience for them—there is always the chance of something going wrong, and at home they are not surrounded by medical staff. Essentially, renal patients are overworked, stressed, and fatigued due to their illness and its invasive treatment, so they do not have the time, energy or enthusiasm to keep video/paper diaries. This meant that video/paper diaries were not well suited to be a staple source of data on participants' interactions with the technology in this context. Such tools can be valuable when working with people with less demanding conditions, or in less intimate spaces; however, for the purposes of our study, being sensitive to the situations of participants was an over-riding consideration that shaped data gathering.

11.3.2   ISSUES WITH OTHER DATA GATHERING METHODS

During the preliminary study, observations tended to be unpredictable in duration and frequency, and it was not possible to conduct observations in a structured way, e.g., using process diagrams or observations sheets. This was because participants had different preferences for when they were willing to be observed, which could be at different stages of dialysis preparation and treatment. Also, when I visited some participants, they had already performed some steps of the preparation (contrary to what we had agreed on the phone). It was therefore not practically possible to observe them throughout the whole treatment from beginning to end; rather, observations of actual interactions were more opportunistic in nature. This meant that observations were not well suited to be a staple source of data on patients' interaction strategies with the technology either.

It was not possible to get access to the home haemodialysis machines to do bench tests, and additionally, since the participants used one of three different machines, it would have been even more impractical to do so. Also, it was not possible to get access to institutional data on actual incidents. When technicians get calls from patients, they record the call on a form, which does not get computerised. For me to get access to these forms, staff members would have to manually photocopy the forms, anonymise them, and send them to me, making this an impractical source of data.

The fact that the participants of the preliminary study used three different machines with different operating procedures, and had been trained by different nurses with different procedures for using their machine, coupled with the fact that the dialysis treatment is complex, made the consultation of device manuals impractical. Therefore, the possibility to compare actual behaviour with prescribed behaviour by referring to the content of device manuals was limited in practice. The most substantial source of data for understanding prescribed behaviour came from the interview with the home nurse, and the most substantial source of data for understanding actual behaviour came from interviews with patients and carers.

11.3.3   INTERVIEWS AS THE STAPLE SOURCE OF DATA

I was able to gather data through a combination of consulting existing dialysis charts, conducting short observations, taking still pictures of the physical environment and of artefacts, and interviewing participants about their experiences of using the technology. Semi-structured interviews proved to be the most substantial source of data, especially with the use of the critical incident technique. The critical incident technique is defined as a "set of procedures for collecting direct observations of human behaviour in such a way as to facilitate their potential usefulness in solving practical problems" (Flanagan, 1954). Typically, a participant is asked to recount experiences they have had. I encountered some challenges when interviewing participants, and the critical incident technique helped to get around these challenges.

11.3.4 CHALLENGES OF INTERVIEWING PATIENTS AND CARERS

The first challenge is that, in such a setting, where the technology is life-sustaining, there is naturally a very high acceptance of the technology, regardless of any design flaws it may have: the interaction difficulties a patient or carer might face while using the technology are peripheral from their perspective, in fact so peripheral that they might not mention them at all. Whilst some patients may be open to having a constructive dialogue about the technology, this is challenging for others. It requires a significant amount of skill for the researcher to determine how far to probe to ensure that the patient does not lose confidence since they depend on the technology for staying alive. The second challenge is that some patients and carers are grateful to have the technology at all in their homes, which makes their lives much easier than having to go to the dialysis unit. Consequently, they may have an inclination to "protect" the system (technology, technicians, nurses, etc.) that makes this possible for them; they would not want either other people in the system or the technology to be seen in a bad light. This can make involving them in critiquing the technology even more problematic. Thirdly, for patients and carers, there is not necessarily a distinction between what constitutes a design flaw and what constitutes a "lack of competency" from the user. On some occasions, patients seemed to want to ensure that they were perceived as being capable of fully handling the machine. This might be either a matter of pride or a matter of ensuring that they were perceived as possessing the required competencies for conducting their treatment independently; after all, they had been formally assessed on this before being allowed to start home haemodialysis treatment. This means that they may be guarded in critiquing the technology, as any critique could be perceived as a lack of competency on their part. Finally, it may be tricky for a patient or carer, who may not be acquainted with HCI or the concept of usability, to understand the motivation behind the study.

11.3.5 THE CRITICAL INCIDENT TECHNIQUE

As a researcher, it was important to recognise the sensitivities of participants' relationships with their (life-saving) technologies and their vulnerabilities. The critical incident technique helped to encourage people to talk openly about some of the challenges they faced. It was helpful in the interviews by, firstly, giving a clear focus to the interview that participants could understand, i.e. incidents they had had with the technology, and secondly, by making clear actual facts (incidents) from participants' more general opinions and impressions, which may be biased for the reasons described above.

During an interview, I prompted the participant to elaborate on incidents they had had, and from this I identified underlying interaction issues. For example, one particular patient mentioned that in the past he occasionally forgot to inject anti-coagulant into the dialysis circuit before starting dialysis. This resulted in blood clotting in the circuit and him having to scrap everything and start his dialysis session from scratch: "I had some er...let's say incidents...once I had to change the line again, because I forgot to take the heparin, and in about one and a half or two hours it started to alarm, because it started clotting, and blood pressure, the pressure in the line goes high and it's alarming and stopping every time." This incident points to the interaction design issue of how to ensure that the patient injects the anti-coagulant. He then explained how he now copes with his issue. He lays out everything he needs to use on a table next to him, so that, on seeing the anti-coagulant bottle there, he remembers to inject it: "before connection and lining the machine, you put everything on the table that you need for this dialysis. When you are connected, on the table should be left the heparin" (the heparin is injected after the patient is connected to the circuit, before starting the treatment on the machine). He added that on one occasion, a random item on the table occluded the anti-coagulant from his line of sight and he forgot to inject it: "I put it on the table, but...because I got something else on the table too...I just couldn't see it at the time when it was needed." This incident points to a vulnerability in his current strategy for coping with the issue. By prompting participants to talk about their incidents in this manner, I was able to identify interaction design issues, participants' strategies for coping with them, and potential vulnerabilities in these strategies. Based on these, we can reflect on design implications.

11.4   CONCLUSIONS

By adapting our approach to what works in practice, we were able to gather data on renal patients' and carers' interactions with dialysis technology. The preliminary study was essential, as it allowed us to gauge the effectiveness of different data gathering techniques. Interviews proved to be the most substantial source of data, and the critical incident technique helped to get around the challenges of interviewing patients/carers in the context of home haemodialysis. Further advice on data gathering is given in Volume 2: Chapter 4.

ACKNOWLEDGEMENTS

We are grateful to all participants for the time, expertise, and experiences they shared with us, and to hospital staff members for facilitating the research. This research is funded by the UK Engineering and Physical Sciences Research Council grant EP/G059063/1.

CHAPTER 12

Experiences in HCI, Healthcare, and Development: Lessons from the PartoPen Project in Kenya

Heather Underwood

This chapter discusses field experiences and lessons learned in the context of the PartoPen case study—a digital pen project designed to improve maternal labour monitoring in developing countries. Three lessons or guidelines are discussed in this chapter based on the fieldwork experiences of the project. Each guideline is followed by action-oriented steps for increasing the likelihood of project success in similar environmental contexts. This chapter offers guidance in the following areas:

- The challenges and importance of time management in healthcare studies;

- Contributing and adding value in addition to conducting healthcare technology research; and

- Balancing emotional attachments to the project with the needs and input of your study participants.

12.1 RESEARCH FOCUS

In 2010 the World Health Organization (WHO) estimated that 287,000 women die every year due to pregnancy-related complications (WHO, 2010). The vast majority (99%) of annual maternal deaths occur in developing countries. Many of these deaths can be prevented with skilled care before, during, and after childbirth (WHO, 2010). The WHO widely promotes the use of a paper-based labour-monitoring tool, the partograph, which was developed in the early 1970s. The partograph facilitates the tracking of maternal condition, fetal condition, and cervical dilation versus time. Used correctly, the partograph can serve as a tool for early detection of serious maternal and fetal complications during labour. However, the partograph is often used incorrectly due to a lack of training and continuing education, and limited resources (Lawn, 2006; Levin, 2011;

Lavender, et al., 2011). The PartoPen[4] research focuses on improving the quality and consistency of maternal labour monitoring in developing countries by promoting better use of the partograph form. The PartoPen provides real-time decision support, audio instructions on correct partograph use, and time-based reminders to support timely patient care. All of the PartoPen functionality is available using only the programmed digital pen and the paper partograph form.

12.1.1 PARTOPEN SPECIFICATIONS AND TECHNICAL DETAILS

The current implementation of the PartoPen system uses the Livescribe[5] 2GB Echo digital pen, which can capture and synchronise audio and handwritten text, and digitise handwritten notes into searchable and printable PDF documents. These pens use an infrared camera in the tip of the pen to capture microdots printed on the paper. The pen can then perform location-specific functions, such as play an instruction prompt when an instruction button is tapped or trigger a decision-support prompt when a nurse plots a measurement indicating abnormal labour. The digital pens are equipped with a speaker, a microphone, a 3.5 mm audio headphone jack, up to 8GB of memory storage (approximately 800 h of audio recording storage), an OLED display, a rechargeable lithium-ion battery, and a micro-USB connector. The PartoPen does not require network connectivity, and can be charged using a micro-USB cell phone charger. The dot pattern can be printed on regular printer paper using a 600 dpi laser printer. The PartoPen is low cost, durable, consumes very little power, requires minimal training, and enhances—rather than replaces—the existing paper partograph.

12.2 STUDY DESIGN: THE PARTOPEN IN KENYA

In March 2012, I spent a week at Kenyatta National Hospital (KNH) in Nairobi, Kenya, observing the labour ward, talking with the nurses, and doing initial usability assessments of the PartoPen system. Kenya was chosen as the study site for the PartoPen project primarily because of the long history of partograph use in the country, which dates back to 1987 when the partograph was introduced to a global audience at the Safe Motherhood Conference in Nairobi. In addition, many of the studies examining barriers to partograph use have been conducted at KNH and surrounding hospitals, which made these facilities a good candidate for evaluating the impact of the PartoPen on known barriers to partograph use. During the visit in March I spent approximately 5–10 h in the labour ward each day taking vigorous notes, learning the processes, and establishing relationships with labour ward staff and hospital administration. In July and August of 2012, I returned to Kenya to implement PartoPen beta at KNH. This study evaluated partograph completion rates for the month immediately prior to the introduction of the PartoPen, and for the month when the PartoPen was in use. "Completion" was measured using a partograph completion rubric previously

---

[4] http://www.partopen.com/
[5] http://www.livescribe.com/

developed by KNH staff for hospital administrative purposes. According to this rubric, a complete partograph has measurements for all of the partograph form sections, and a complete labour summary. A research assistant scanned the 369 partograph forms completed in the month prior to PartoPen introduction. During the month of PartoPen use, 457 partograph forms were collected.

12.3 STUDY EXPERIENCE: LESSONS LEARNED

The PartoPen case study illustrates a before-and-after intervention at a labour ward in Kenya. Approximately 50 nurses participated in the two-month study. During the study, I derived several "rules of thumb" from my experience. The guidelines outlined in this section are intended to be generalizable to most HCI work in healthcare settings, while being supported by specific examples from the PartoPen case study. I have also described several actionable strategies I found useful for putting these lessons into practice throughout the research process. Preparing for fieldwork, and implementing these strategies is part of the larger concept of "readying the researcher," which is elaborated on in Volume 2: Chapter 2.

12.3.1 LESSON 1: TIME MANAGEMENT

Lesson 1 is a reminder that researchers need to make time to be patient. It is difficult to ask research participants, especially busy nurses in understaffed hospitals, to take an hour or two to talk with you about your project (which they may or may not have any interest or investment in whatsoever). However, if you make yourself available and present, it will not take as long as you think for people to start asking you questions, and become interested in what you are doing in their hospital. It is common for researchers to believe that budgeting time for "sitting around" is not going to pay off in terms of their grant obligations or deliverable deadlines. However, if you do not make the initial investment in your participants and the environment in which they work, you usually have lost sight of the larger goal altogether. So scale your study to account for this necessary investment while still staying true to deadlines and financial constraints.

Budgeting extra time—a three-month trip to Kenya instead of a one-month trip—proved invaluable to the PartoPen project. I used the extra time to accomplish many things, including administrative tasks that were simplified by being there in person. I spent most of my time in the labour ward with nurses, talking with them, helping them perform patient in-take when staff numbers were low, and asking questions when time permitted. One of the benefits of the PartoPen project is that the pen itself is low profile, and a valuable research and note-taking tool in and of itself. When I spent time in the labour ward, I would use a digital pen to write down observations and take notes. Simply using the pen in front of the nurses drew their attention, caused them to ask a number of insightful questions, and illustrated the simplicity and broad use cases of the pen. By using the pen, I was able to decrease the perception of additional work often associated with the introduction of a new technology. Although it seemed like I was just 'sitting around' taking notes, it promoted communication and interest in the project.

During the three weeks I spent observing and interacting with the staff prior to the start of the study, I tasked myself with finding out three things about each nurse beyond obvious demographic characteristics. Discovering these things about each nurse allowed me to better understand their values and incentive systems. For example, during an afternoon tea break (which I have found is the optimal time for getting to know your study participants and getting answers to your questions) I spoke with a nurse who eventually told me: "The pen needs a cap! I don't have time to wash my uniform every night and the pen marks are hard to get out! If you do my laundry, I'll use it." Most of the nurses who work at KNH live about two hours, by bus, away from the hospital, which means that in addition to their 8–12 h shifts, they are stuck in traffic for another 4 h. Adding makeshift caps to the pens noticeably shifted the mood among the nurses. By learning where the nurses lived and how they commuted to work each day I discovered an underlying problem with the design of the system, addressed it, and did not infringe on one of the things they truly value: their time.

12.3.2 LESSON 2: DOING MORE THAN THE RESEARCH REQUIRES

The second lesson refers to helping your study participants in an immediate way, regardless of whether providing that help falls in line with your overall research agenda. By spending time with research participants, asking questions, and observing the environment in which you will be conducting your research, you will begin to understand the necessary skills for completing various tasks. Undoubtedly, there will be tasks that you are capable of doing given your current skills. By offering immediate assistance with tasks you are qualified to do, you accomplish several things. First, you illustrate your competence to the people you will be working with. Second, by learning to do the work that your research participants do every day, you will develop respect for them and the specific skills they have. Also, by successfully doing some of the work that they do every day, you will gain participants' trust. Third, by actually performing various tasks within the healthcare setting, you develop an intimate knowledge of detailed processes that often seem obscure when observed from the outside. Deep knowledge of specific processes within the clinic will allow you to gain a more complete picture of problems and areas for improvement that your research may be able to directly address. Finally, by keeping lesson 2 in mind, you will keep lesson 1 in check. Getting to know your participants, and spending a great deal of time in the environment you are working in, accomplishes many things; however, if you are not providing any valuable service or insight for long periods of time, there is a strong possibility that you will become a harmful distraction or an annoying, question-asking obstacle for people trying to do their work. By becoming a valuable contributor within the existing clinical workflow, you will be able to learn about your participants in an interactive way on a level playing field and help them with their work instead of getting in their way.

My first extended visit to KNH in March 2012 was intended to be a trip solely for observation. On the first day, no one seemed interested in me or why I was there. Three hours went by, and a few nurses had said "hello." One nurse brought me tea around noon. On the second day, I returned to the labour ward and everyone seemed surprised to see me. Now, I realize that this is a very common occurrence—they do not expect you to come back. It makes sense in a place where so many non-governmental organisations (NGOs), donors, and researchers come and go, promising changes, and failing to deliver; trust takes time and follow-through to develop.

The initial lack of communication, and my unfamiliarity with the terminology of the labour ward made it difficult to understand labour ward processes. I started writing down all the words I did not know, and asked during tea breaks what they meant. By the end of the week, I was helping with patient intake, making patient files with all of the appropriate forms, and occasionally answering the phone (my Swahili was getting pretty good at this point). It was much easier to pinpoint where I could add immediate value for the nurses once I understood the medical language they were speaking. Creating a dictionary is a valuable tool that can simplify your research and contribute to your unique and highly specific understanding of the issues you are interested in.

In cases where it is not as clear where you can provide value, two things will always apply. First, show up. This is applicable to every HCI research area in any part of the world. Second, in healthcare there are always patients and staff who can use a little assistance or a kind word of encouragement. Both are powerful illustrations of commitment and humility—two characteristics that will accelerate your research and remind you of the underlying reasons you do the work you do.

12.3.3 LESSON 3: A LESSON IN HUMILITY

In healthcare, where patients' lives are often at stake, there is no amount of financial constraints or donor expectations or deadlines that will justify your research negatively impacting the health and wellbeing of your research subjects. The growing number of FailFaires[6] and papers documenting the failures of development projects indicates the gradually shifting culture, which values "do no harm" policies over data collection at all costs. Entering a healthcare setting should be a humbling experience, and if you do not check your ego at the door, it will not be long before it gets checked for you.

I learned early in the PartoPen project that it is detrimental to associate yourself so closely with your research that everything becomes personal. During my initial usability tests in March 2012, several aspects of the PartoPen functionality were underscored as clearly unusable. In the first iteration of the PartoPen project, the pen emitted audio when a nurse recorded an alarming measurement. The audio was recorded in my voice and was only played once. The first nurse to use the pen said something along the lines of "I can't understand a word this thing is saying…and I think what it said was wrong!" My first impulse was to retort, "It's not wrong! That's exactly what the WHO user manual on partograph use says! And I spoke so clearly and slowly; how can it be

---

[6] http://failfaire.org/about/

hard to understand what I was saying?" This is obviously the wrong response. Ego slightly bruised, I returned to the drawing board that night, and realised that the WHO manual was in fact inaccurate given the current version of the partograph that nurses were using. In addition, it became clear that it was difficult for the nurses to understand my voice even without it being recorded on the pen. I changed the audio prompts to text on the pen's display, accompanied by a ring-tone from the pen's speaker. The new design was well received, and the nurses expressed their appreciation for the quick fix. Seeing the quick change based on their feedback also encouraged the nurses to suggest other design changes and be more vocal and honest about the project.

In an academic environment like graduate school, it is easy to become convinced that the important deliverables are publications with real data and statistical analysis, convincing answers to all of the questions committee members could possibly ask, and "expert" status in the microscopic body of knowledge you produce. However, I find it useful to make a second list, which helps me balance the urgency to complete academic requirements with the realities of my fieldwork environment. My list usually contains things that I will personally feel a sense of accomplishment for completing. The first iteration of my personal PartoPen list included: know all of the nurses' names by the time I leave; practice my Swahili even though everyone speaks English; and do not faint in the delivery room. The second iteration was more specific and included performing specific project-related tasks like buying and installing a new printer and supplying it with ink and paper; capacity-building activities like teaching IT staff how to program the digital pens and collect data; and personal goals like trying out recipes the nurses gave me, and printing pictures of the nurses for them. Very few of the things on these lists, if performed in isolation, would contribute to writing my dissertation or publishing my next paper; however, by doing the things on this list, I never found myself in a situation where getting the data at all costs was the only thing that defined my work.

12.4   CONCLUSIONS

When I left Kenya in August 2012 I had collected 2 months of partographs, 50 surveys, and 2 notebooks of qualitative observations. More notably, the labour ward at KNH continued the use of the PartoPen system, which is currently run and managed entirely by hospital staff and labour ward nurses. Continuing to follow the lessons discussed in this paper, I have been able to create a system that fits the needs of the labour ward staff without introducing extra work, training, or financial burdens. A recent letter from KNH administration praised the PartoPen system for improving the number of completed partographs in patient files, and higher quality patient care due to increased awareness of labour monitoring practices. The current success of the PartoPen project is largely due to the genuine relationships I was able to develop during my fieldwork by showing up, being useful, and quickly responding to feedback without taking the critiques personally.

By budgeting more time than you think you will need, providing tangible value when you are qualified to do so, and keeping your pride in perspective, you will be more prepared to deal with the many unanticipated and subtle aspects of doing HCI research in the highly sensitive field of healthcare. The second volume of this guidebook builds on the experiences and advice given here and provides an applicable set of guidelines for HCI fieldwork in healthcare.

ACKNOWLEDGEMENTS

The PartoPen research is supported by the ATLAS Institute at the University of Colorado Boulder, an NSF Graduate Research Fellowship, and a Gates Grand Challenge Explorations grant. I would also like to thank the nurses and staff at Kenyatta National Hospital, and Dr. John Ong'ech, who championed the PartoPen project in Kenya.

References

Barach P. and Weinger, M. B. (2007). Trauma Team Performance. In W. C. Wilson, C. M. Grande, and D. B. Hoyt (Eds.), *Trauma: Emergency Resuscitation, Perioperative Anesthesia, Surgical Management*, Informa Healthcare USA, Inc., New York, NY, 101-113. DOI: 10.3109/9781420052442-7.

Bardram, J. E. (1997, November). I Love the System—I Just Don't Use It! *Proceedings of the international ACM SIGGROUP conference on supporting group work: the integration challenge* (pp. 251-260). ACM. DOI: 10.1145/266838.266922.

Bardram, J. E., Frost, M., Szanto, K., and Marcu, G. (2012). The MONARCA Self-Assessment System: A Persuasive Personal Monitoring System for Bipolar Patients. *Proceedings of the 2nd ACM SIGHIT International Health Informatics Symposium, IHI'12* (pp. 21–30). New York: ACM. DOI: 10.1145/2110363.2110370. DOI: http://dl.acm.org/citation.cfm?doid=2110363.2110370.

Beach, C., Croskerry, P., and Shapiro, M. (2003). Profiles in Patient Safety: Emergency Care Transitions. *Academic Emergency Medicine*, 10(4), 364-367. DOI: 10.1111/j.1553-2712.2003.tb01350.x.

Behara, R., Wears, R. L., Perry, S., Eisenberg, E., Murphy, L., Vanderhoef, Shapiro, M., Beach, C., Croskerry, P., and Cosby, K. (2005). A Conceptual Framework for Studying the Safety of Transitions in Emergency Care. In K. Henriksen, J. B. Battles, E. S. Marks and D. I. Lewin (Eds.), *Advances in Patient Safety: From Research to Implementation, Volume 2: Concepts and Methodology* (http://www.ahrq.gov/downloads/pub/advances/vol2/Behara.pdf ed., pp. 21). Rockville, MD: Agency for Healthcare Research and Quality (US).

Berg, M., Aarts, J., and van der Lei, J. (2003). ICT in Health Care: Sociotechnical Approaches. *Methods of Information in Medicine*, 42(4), 297–301.

Beyer, H. and Holtzblatt, K. (1998). *Contextual Design: Defining Customer Centred Systems*. San Francisco, CA: Morgan Kaufmann Publishers. DOI: http://dl.acm.org/citation.cfm?id=291229.

Blandford, A., Adams, A., and Furniss, D. (2009). Understanding the Situated Use of Healthcare Technologies. *Proc. CHI 2009 Workshop on Evaluating New Interactions in Healthcare*, ACM Press, 1–4.

Bødker, S., Ehn, P., Sjögren, D., and Sundblad, Y. (2000). "Co-operative Design – Perspectives on 20 Years with 'the Scandinavian IT Design Model'", *Proc. NordiCHI.*

Braun, V. and Clarke, V. (2006). Using Thematic Analysis in Psychology. *Qualitative Research in Psychology,* 3(2), 77–101. DOI: 10.1191/1478088706qp063oa.

Calnan, M., Almond, S., and Smith, N. (2003). Ageing and Public Satisfaction with the Health Service: An Analysis of Recent Trends. *Social Science & Medicine,* 57(4), 757–762. DOI: 10.1016/s0277-9536(03)00128-x.

Chan A. J., Islam M. K., Rosewall T., Jaffray D. A., Easty A. C., and Cafazzo J. A. (2010). The Use of Human Factors Methods to Identify and Mitigate Safety Issues in Radiation Therapy. *Radiother Oncol.* Dec; 97(3):596–600. DOI: 10.1016/j.radonc.2010.09.026.

Charmaz, K. (2006). *Constructing Grounded Theory: A Practical Guide through Qualitative Analysis.* Thousand Oaks, CA: Sage.

Chilvers, J., Thomas, C., and Stanbury, A. (2011). The Impact of a Ward-Based Mindfulness Programme on Recorded Aggression in a Medium Secure Facility for Women with Learning Disabilities. *Journal of Learning Disability and Offending Behavior,* 2, 1, 27–41. DOI: 10.5042/jldob.2011.0026.

Cohen, M. D., and Hilligoss, B. (2010). The Published Literature on Handoffs in Hospitals: Deficiencies Identified in an Extensive Review. *Quality & Safety in Health Care,* 19(6), 493–497. DOI: 10.1136/qshc.2009.033480.

Coiera, E. (2007). "Putting the Technical Back into Socio-Technical Systems Research," *International Journal of Medical Informatics* 76, S1, pp. S98–S103. DOI: 10.1016/j.ijmed-inf.2006.05.026.

Dowding, D., Mitchell, N., Randell, R., Foster, R., Lattimer, V., and Thompson, C. (2009). Nurses' Use of Computerised Clinical Decision Support Systems: A Case Site Analysis. *Journal of Clinical Nursing,* 18, 1159–1167. DOI: 10.1111/j.1365-2702.2008.02607.x.

Emerson, R., Fretz, R., and Shaw, L. (1995). *Writing Ethnographic Fieldnotes.* Chicago: University of Chicago Press. DOI: 10.7208/chicago/9780226206851.001.0001.

Flanagan, J. C. (1954). The Critical Incident Technique. *Psychological Bulletin,* 51(4), 327. DOI: 10.1037/h0061470.

Frost, M., Doryab, A., and Bardram, J. E. (2013). Supporting Disease Insight through Data Analysis: Refinements of the MONARCA Self-Assessment System. *Ubicomp '13 The 2013 ACM Conference on Ubiquitous Computing.* New York, NY, USA: ACM. DOI: 10.1145/2493432.2493507.

Frykholm, O., Nilsson, M., Groth, K. and Yngling, A. (2012). Interaction Design in a Complex Context: Medical Multi-Disciplinary Team Meetings. *Proc. NordiChi*. DOI: 10.1145/2399016.2399070.

Frykholm, O., Lantz, A., Groth, K. and Walldius, Å. (2010). Medicine Meets Engineering in Cooperative Design of Collaborative Decision-Supportive System. *Proc. CBMS*. DOI:10.1109/CBMS.2010.6042625.

Gelbart, B., Barfield, C., and Watkins, A. (2009). Ethical and Legal Considerations in Video Recording Neonatal Resuscitations. *Journal of Medical Ethics*, 35(2), 120–124. DOI: 10.1136/jme.2008.024612.

Gilbert, K. (Ed.) (2001). *The Emotional Nature of Qualitative Research*. CRC Press.

Glaser, B. G. and Strauss, A. L. (1967). *The Discovery of Grounded Theory: Strategies for Qualitative Research*. New York: Aldine Publishing Company.

Greenbaum J. and Kyng, M. (1992). *Design at Work: Cooperative Design of Computer Systems*, Lawrence Erlbaum Associates, Inc.

Hammersley, M. and Atkinson, P. (1995). *Ethnography: Principles in Practice*. London: Routledge.

Health and Human Services Secretary's Advisory Committee on Human Research Protections. (January 2008). Summary letter available online at http://www.hhs.gov/ohrp/sachrp/sachrpletter013108.html.

Hedican, E. J. (2006). Understanding Emotional Experience in Fieldwork: Responding to Grief in a Northern Aboriginal Village. *International Journal of Qualitative Methods*, 5(1) Retrieved January 8 2013 from http://www.ualberta.ca/~iiqm/backissues/5_1/pdf/hedican.pdf.

Horwitz, L., Meredith, T., Schuur, J. D., Shah, N. R., Kulkarni, R. G., and Jenq, G. Y. (2009). Dropping the Baton: A Qualitative Analysis of Failures During the Transition from Emergency Department to Inpatient Care. *Annals of Emergency Medicine*, 53(6), 701–710. DOI: 10.1016/j.annemergmed.2008.05.007.

Hughes, J. A, Randall, D., and Shapiro, D. (1992). "Faltering from Ethnography to Design." *Proceedings of the 1992 ACM conference on Computer-supported cooperative work*, Pages 115-122. DOI: 10.1145/143457.143469.

Hutchinson, M., Vickers, M., Jackson, D., and Wilkes, L. (2006). Workplace Bullying in Nursing: Towards a More Critical Organisational Perspective. *Nursing Inquiry*, 13(2), 118–126. DOI: 10.1111/j.1440-1800.2006.00314.x.

Jaspers, M. W., Peute, L. W., Lauteslager, A., and Bakker, P. J. (2008). Pre-Post Evaluation of Physicians' Satisfaction with a Redesigned Electronic Medical Record System. *Studies in health technology and informatics*, 136, 303.

Junior Doctors Committee. (2004). *Safe Handover: Safe Patients*. London: British Medical Association.

Kane, B., Groth, K., and Randall, D. (2011). Special issue on Medical Team Meetings. *Behaviour and Information Technology*, 30(4).

Kvale, S. (1996). *Interviews: An introduction to qualitative research interviewing*, London: Sage.

Lavender, T., Omoni, G., Lee, K., Wakasiaka, S., et al. (2011). Students' Experiences of Using the Partograph in Kenyan Labour Wards. *African Journal of Midwifery and Women's Health* 5, 3, 117–122.

Lawn, J. and Kerber, K. (2006). *Opportunities for Africa's Newborns: Practical Data, Policy and Programmatic Support for Newborn Care in Africa*. Geneva: World Health Organization.

Leonard, M., Graham, S., and Bonacum, D. (2004). The Human Factor: The Critical Importance of Effective Teamwork and Communication in Providing Safe Care. *Quality and Safety in Health Care*, 13 (Suppl 1). DOI: 10.1136/qshc.2004.010033.

Levin, L. (2011). Use of the Partograph: Effectiveness, Training, Modifications, and Barriers. *A Literature Review. Agency for International Development, Fistula Care, EngenderHealth* 28.

Lieb, K. (2004). Borderline Personality Disorder. *Lancet* 364, 53–461. DOI: 10.1016/S0140-6736(04)16770-6.

Linehan, M. M. (1993). *Skills Training Manual for Treating Borderline Personality Disorder*. Guildford.

Marcu, G., Bardram, J. E., and Gabrielli, S. (2011). A Framework for Overcoming Challenges in Designing Persuasive Monitoring Systems for Mental Illness. *Proceedings of Pervasive Health 2011* (pp. 1–8). Dublin, Ireland: IEEE Xplore.

Mackenzie, C. F., Xiao, Y., Hu, F. M., Seagull, F. J., and Fitzgerald, M. (2007). Video as a Tool for Improving Tracheal Intubation Tasks for Emergency Medical and Trauma Care. *Annals of emergency medicine*, 50(4), 436–442. DOI: 10.1016/j.annemergmed.2007.06.487.

McDonald, S. (2005). Studying Actions in Context: A Qualitative Shadowing Method for Organizational Research. *Qualitative Research*, 5(4), 455–473. DOI: 10.1177/1468794105056923.

Monahan, T and Fisher, J. A. (2010). Benefits of 'Observer Effects': Lessons from the Field. *Qualitative Research*. 2010 vol 10(3) 357–376. DOI: 10.1177/1468794110362874

Noy, C. (2008). Sampling Knowledge: The Hermeneutics of Snowball Sampling in Qualitative Research. *International Journal of Social Research Methodology*, 11(4), 327–344. DOI: 10.1080/13645570701401305.

Olwal, A., Frykholm, O., Groth, K., and Moll, J. (2011). Exploring the Potential for Collaborative Interaction in Medical Team Meetings. *Proc. INTERACT*.

Øvretveit, J.(1992). *Health Services Quality*, Oxford: Blackwell.

Randell, R., Wilson, S., and Woodward, P. (2011a). The Importance of the Verbal Shift Handover Report: A Multi-Site Case Study. *International Journal of Medical Informatics*, 80(11), 803–812. DOI: 10.1016/j.ijmedinf.2011.08.006.

Randell, R., Wilson, S., and Woodward, P. (2011b). Variations and Commonalities in Processes of Collaboration: The Need for Multi-Site Workplace Studies. *Journal of Computer Supported Cooperative Work*, 20, 37–59. DOI: 10.1007/s10606-010-9127-6.

Randell, R., Wilson, S., Woodward, P., and Galliers, J. (2010). Beyond Handover: Supporting Awareness for Continuous Coverage. *Cognition, Technology & Work*. DOI: 10.1007/s10111-010-0138-3.

Randell, R., Wilson, S., Woodward, P., and Galliers, J. (2011). The ConStratO Model of Handover: A Tool to Support Technology Design and Evaluation. *Behaviour & Information Technology*, 30(4), 489–498. DOI: 10.1080/0144929x.2010.547220.

Robertson, B. (2011). The Adaption and Application of Mindfulness-Based Psychotherapeutic Oractices for Individuals with Intellectual Disabilities. *Advances in Mental Health and Intellectual Disabilities* 5, 5, 46–52. DOI: 10.1108/20441281111180664.

Rode, J. A. (2011, May). Reflexivity in Digital Anthropology. *Proceedings of the SIGCHI Conference on Human Factors in Computing Systems* (pp. 123–132). ACM. DOI: 10.1145/1978942.1978961.

Ruhstaller, T., Roe, H., Thürlimann, B., and Nicholl, J. J. (2006). The Multidisciplinary Meeting: An Indispensable Aid to Communication between Different Specialties. *European Journal of Cancer*, 42:2459–2462. DOI: 10.1016/j.ejca.2006.03.034.

Russell, C. (1999). Interviewing Vulnerable Old People: Ethical and Methodological Implications of Imagining Our Subjects. *Journal of Aging Studies*, 13(4), 403-417. DOI: 10.1016/S0890-4065(99)00018-3.

Sallnäs, E.-L., Moll, J., Frykholm, O., Groth, K., and Forsslund, J. (2011). Pointing in Multi-Disciplinary Medical Meetings. *Proc. CBMS*. DOI: 10.1109/CBMS.2011.5999133.

Sellen, K., Chignell, M., Straus, S., Callum, J., Pendergrast, J., and Halliday, A. (2010). Using Motion Sensing to Study Human Computer Interaction in Hospital Settings. *Proceedings of international ACM conference on Measuring Behavior* (pp.297–300). ACM.

Thieme, A., Wallace, J., Johnson, P., Lindley, S., McCarthy, J., Olivier, P., and Meyer, T. D. (2012). Can We Introduce Mindfulness Practice through Digital Design? *Proc. BCS HCI* 2012, http://ewic.bcs.org/content/ConWebDoc/48799.

Thieme, A., Wallace, J., Johnson, P., McCarthy, J., Lindley, S., Wright, P., Olivier, P., and Meyer, T. D. (2013). Design to Promote Mindfulness Practice and Sense of Self for Vulnerable Women in Secure Hospital Services. *Proc. CHI* 2013, 2647–2656. DOI: 10.1145/2470654.2481366.

Van de Ven, A. H. (2007). *Engaged Scholarship: A Guide for Organizational and Social Research*. Oxford: Oxford University Press.

Wears, R. L. (2012). Poverty amid Plenty. *BMJ Quality & Safety*, 21(7), 533–534. DOI: 10.1136/bmjqs-2012-000916.

Wilson, S., Randell, R., Galliers, J., and Woodward, P. (2009). Reconceptualising Clinical Handover: Information Sharing for Situation Awareness. Paper presented at the European Conference on Cognitive Ergonomics Otaniemi, Helsinki metropolitan area, Finland.

World Health Organization. (2010). Fact Sheet. http://www.who.int/mediacentre/factsheets/fs348/en/index.html.

Yen, S., Zlotnick, C. and Costello, E. (2002). Affect Regulation in Women with Borderline Personality Disorder Traits. *The Journal of Nervous and Mental Disease* 100, 10, 693–696. DOI: 10.1097/00005053-200210000-00006.

Yin, R. K. (2003). *Case Study Research: Design and Methods* (3rd ed.). Thousand Oaks, California: Sage Publications.

Zheng, K., Padman, R., Johnson, M. P., and Diamond, H. S. (2005). Understanding Technology Adoption in Clinical Care: Clinician Adoption Behavior of a Point-of-Care Reminder System. *International journal of medical informatics*, 74(7), 535–543. DOI: 10.1016/j.ijmedinf.2005.03.007.

Biographies

EDITOR BIOGRAPHIES

Dominic Furniss is a Researcher Co-Investigator on the CHI+MED project at University College London. He investigates the design and use of medical devices in hospitals. His interests include the development of theory to support the understanding of performance in socio-technical systems. He is the lead editor and also the author of Chapter 3.

Address: UCL Interaction Centre, University College London, Gower Street, London WC1E 6BT, U.K.

Aisling Ann O'Kane is a Ph.D. student on the CHI+MED project at University College London. Her research is on the situated use of mobile medical technologies by patients. Her interests include the connections between human factors engineering and user experience. She is a co-editor.

Address: UCL Interaction Centre, University College London, Gower Street, London WC1E 6BT, U.K.

Rebecca Randell is a Senior Translational Research Fellow in the School of Healthcare, University of Leeds, where she leads the decision-making research theme. Her research focuses on studying how technology impacts the decision making of healthcare professionals. She is a co-editor and also the author of Chapter 5.

Address: School of Healthcare, University of Leeds, Leeds LS2 9UT, U.K.

Svetlena Taneva is a Human Factors Specialist at Healthcare Human Factors, UHN. Svetlena specializes in the development and evaluation of technology and organizational processes for clinical environments. For the past eight years, Svetlena worked and published extensively in the area of HCI in healthcare. She is a co-editor and also a co-author of Chapter 4.

Address: Healthcare Human Factors, University Health Network, 190 Elizabeth Street, Toronto, ON M5G 2C4.

Helena Mentis is an Assistant Professor in the Department of Information Systems at the University of Maryland, Baltimore County. She examines the challenges clinical healthcare providers face in the embodied sharing and understanding of ambiguous and interpretive health information. She has conducted fieldwork in healthcare in the U.S. and the U.K. She is a co-editor.

Address: Department of Information Systems, University of Maryland, Baltimore County, 1000 Hilltop Circle, Baltimore, MD 21250.

Ann Blandford is Professor of Human–Computer Interaction at UCL, and leads the CHI+MED project on making interactive medical devices safer. Her expertise is in models and methods for studying interactive systems "in the wild", with a particular focus on healthcare. She is the senior editor and a co-author of Chapter 11.

Address: UCL Interaction Centre, University College London, Gower Street, London WC1E 6BT, U.K.

AUTHOR BIOGRAPHIES

Kevin Armour is an award-winning Canadian Industrial Designer working at Healthcare Human Factors, developing medical device interfaces and wearable monitoring devices. Kevin has experience working as a design consultant, developing products for a range of industries, from automotive accessories to home and garden.

Address: Healthcare Human Factors, University Health Network, 190 Elizabeth Street, Toronto, ON M5G 2C4, Canada.

Jeannie L. Callum is director of Transfusion Medicine and Tissue Banks at Sunnybrook Health Sciences Center in Toronto and an associate professor in the Department of Laboratory Medicine and Pathobiology at the University of Toronto. She earned her medical degree and completed a fellowship in internal medicine at the University of Toronto. She is a co-author of Chapter 1.

Address: Sunnybrook Health Sciences Centre, 2075 Bayview Ave, Toronto, ON M4N 3M5, Canada.

Anjum Chagpar is the Managing Director of Healthcare Human Factors, a team of 25 engineers, psychologists, and designers transforming healthcare through the application of Human Factors. Her interests include the design of health technologies for under-served populations as well as emerging economies. She is the lead author of Chapter 4.

Address: Healthcare Human Factors, University Health Network, 190 Elizabeth Street, Toronto, ON M5G 2C4, Canada.

Deborah Chan is a Human Factors Engineer at Healthcare Human Factors, UHN. She has been designing user interfaces for the past 10 years for both public and private sectors. Her focus is the use of human factors methods in the healthcare industry, particularly in the area of cancer care.

Address: Healthcare Human Factors, University Health Network, 190 Elizabeth Street, Toronto, ON M5G 2C4, Canada.

Mark Chignell is Professor of Mechanical and Industrial Engineering and has taught at the University of Toronto since 1990. He is Director of the Interactive Media Laboratory and Director of the Knowledge Media Design Institute. His research is concerned with augmenting human capability through innovative user interface design. He is a co-author of Chapter 1.

Address: Interactive Media Lab, Department of Mechanical and Industrial Engineering, University of Toronto, 5 King's College Road, Toronto, ON, M5S 3G8, Canada.

Mads Frost is a Ph.D. fellow at the IT University of Copenhagen. He investigates the design and use of pervasive personal monitoring systems in healthcare. His interests are awareness and motivation of patients in healthcare systems. He is the lead author of Chapter 8.

Address: Pervasive Interaction Technology (PIT) Lab, IT University of Copenhagen, Rued Langgaards Vej 7, 2300 Copenhagen S, Denmark.

Oscar Frykholm has a Ph.D. in Interaction Design from the Royal Institute of Technology and is working with Interaction Design at Karolinska University Hospital. His main interest is to use prototyping and information visualisation to improve work processes. He is a co-author of Chapter 7.

Address: Innovation Center, Development and Innovation, Karolinska University Hospital, Stockholm, Sweden.

Media Technology and Interaction Design, School of Computer Science and Communication, Royal Institute of Technology, Stockholm, Sweden U.K.

Kristina Groth is associate professor in HCI at the Royal Institute of Technology and responsible for Telemedicine development at Karolinska University hospital. Her research and development work focus on computer-supported collaborative work and mediated communication. She is the lead author of Chapter 7.

Address: Innovation Center, Development and Innovation, Karolinska University Hospital, Stockholm, Sweden.

Media Technology and Interaction Design, School of Computer Science and Communication, Royal Institute of Technology, Stockholm, Sweden U.K.

Alison Halliday, MLT, CTBS is a Senior Technologist in the Blood and Tissue Bank at Sunnybrook Health Sciences Centre. Her primary responsibility is for the Tissue Bank. She is also involved in the implementation and support of the Blood Bank Information System and as a special project implemented the remote fridge system in the Sunnybrook operating room. She is a co-author of Chapter 1.

Address: Sunnybrook Health Sciences Centre, 2075 Bayview Ave, Toronto, ON M4N 3M5, Canada.

Brian Hilligoss is an assistant professor in the College of Public Health at The Ohio State University. He investigates the interplay of organizational routines, communication, and information systems in healthcare. His interests focus on enhancing high reliability in complex socio-technical systems. He is the author of Chapter 6.

Address: College of Public Health, The Ohio State University, 224 Cunz Hall, 1841 Neil Avenue, Columbus, OH 43210, U.S.

Steven Houben is a Ph.D. fellow at the IT University of Copenhagen. His research focuses on activity-centric multi-device information spaces to support the nomadic workflow of clinicians in hospitals. More generally, he is interested in distributed user interface technology, interactive displays, and mobile computing. He is a co-author of Chapter 8.

Address: Pervasive Interaction Technology (PIT) Lab, IT University of Copenhagen, Rued Langgaards Vej 7, 2300 Copenhagen S, Denmark.

Jennifer Jeon is a Human Factors Engineer with Healthcare Human Factors at the University Health Network, Toronto, Canada. Her interests include applications of human factors methods to design and optimize complex systems in healthcare such as computerized physician order entry systems and electronic medical records. She is a co-author of Chapter 4.

Address: Healthcare Human Factors, University Health Network, 190 Elizabeth Street, Toronto, ON M5G 2C4, Canada.

Paula Johnson is the Research & Development Manager within Calderstones Partnership NHS Foundation Trust, a specialist forensic hospital for people with a learning disability. She promotes evidence-based practice and research for patient benefit within the Trust. She is a co-author of Chapter 9.

Address: Calderstones Partnership NHS Foundation Trust, Whalley, Lancashire BB7 9PE, U.K.

Jennifer Martin is Programme Manager of MindTech Healthcare Technology Co-operative. She was previously Senior Research Fellow at Nottingham University investigating the design of medical devices. She currently serves on the Human Factors Committee for the Association of the Advancement of Medical Instrumentation (AAMI). She is a co-author of Chapter 10.

Address: Faculty of Engineering, University of Nottingham, Nottingham, NG7 2RD, U.K.

Astrid Mayer is a medical oncologist with an interest in the use of IT to improve healthcare. She is interested in the development and use of technology empowering patients allowing them to be independent and informing their decision process. Astrid is a collaborator on the CHI+MED project on making medical devices safer. She is a co-author of Chapter 11.

Address: Department of Oncology, Royal Free NHS Trust, Pond Street, London, NW3 2QG, U.K.

Tara McCurdie works with clients in both public and private sectors to address the usability and safety of healthcare technology and workflow in order to reduce preventable patient injuries that can occur during the provision of care. Tara's experience includes procurement decision support, technology assessments, and product and interface design. She is a co-author of Chapter 4.

Address: Healthcare Human Factors, University Health Network, 190 Elizabeth Street, Toronto, ON M5G 2C4, Canada.

Cassie McDaniel worked with the Human Factors team and other designers at UHN to improve technology and healthcare processes for patients and caregivers. Specifically, she worked on user interfaces, user experiences, and medical devices, from medical products to mobile apps.

Address: Healthcare Human Factors, University Health Network, 190 Elizabeth Street, Toronto, ON M5G 2C4, Canada.

Thomas Daniel Meyer is a Senior Lecturer in Clinical Psychology at the Institute of Neuroscience at Newcastle University. He also delivers and provides training in Cognitive Behavioral Therapy. His research focuses on bipolar disorders and the promotion of physical health, psychological wellbeing, and mindfulness, more generally. He is a co-author of Chapter 9.

Address: Institute of Neuroscience, Newcastle University, Newcastle NE1 7RU, U.K.

Patrick Olivier is Professor of Human-Computer Interaction at Newcastle University where he leads Culture Lab's Digital Interaction Group. He is interested in exploring approaches to configuring participatory and experience-centered design activities, in particular in relation to maintenance of the health and wellbeing of vulnerable people. He is a co-author of Chapter 9.

Address: School of Computer Science, Newcastle University, Newcastle NE1 7RU, U.K.

Jacob Pendergrast graduated in 1999 from Dalhousie Medical School and completed his training in internal medicine, hematology, and transfusion medicine at the University of Toronto before taking a staff appointment at the University Health Network, where he serves as an Associate Medical Director of the Blood Transfusion Service. He is a co-author of Chapter 1.

Address: University Health Network, R. Fraser Elliott Building, 190 Elizabeth St., Toronto, ON, M5G 2C4, Canada.

Atish Rajkomar is a Ph.D. student on the CHI+MED project at University College London. His research is on understanding patients' situated interactions with home haemodialysis machines. His interests include the design and evaluation of healthcare socio-technical systems, particularly using cognitive engineering approaches. He is the lead author of Chapter 11.

Address: UCL Interaction Centre, University College London, Gower Street, London WC1E 6BT, U.K.

Aleksandra Sarcevic is an Assistant Professor at the College of Computing and Informatics at Drexel University. Her research interests are in computer supported cooperative work, focusing on ethnographic studies of practice and coordination in high-risk medical settings that inform technology design and implementation. She is the author of Chapter 2.

Address: College of Computing and Informatics, Drexel University, 3141 Chestnut St., Philadelphia, PA 19104, U.S.

Kate Sellen is an Assistant Professor at OCAD University where she teaches human factors. She is interested in understanding adoption and adaptation behaviors to new technology in clinical settings, innovation approaches in healthcare, and the role of design in reducing medical error. She is the lead author of Chapter 1.

Address: OCAD University, Faculty of Design, 205 Richmond St., Toronto, ON, Canada.

Sarah Sharples is a Professor of Human Factors at the University of Nottingham. Her main areas of interest and expertise are Human-Computer Interaction, cognitive ergonomics and development of quantitative and qualitative research methodologies for examination of interaction with innovative technologies in complex systems. She is a co-author of Chapter 10.

Address: Faculty of Engineering, University of Nottingham, Nottingham, NG7 2RD, U.K.

Anja Thieme is a Researcher in Human-Computer Interaction in Culture Lab at Newcastle University. Her research focuses on the design and evaluation of technology to promote the mental health and emotional wellbeing of people who have very complex mental health problems. She is the lead author of Chapter 9.

Address: School of Computer Science, Newcastle University, Newcastle NE1 7RU, U.K.

Ross Thomson is a Ph.D. student on the MATCH project at the University of Nottingham. His research is on home use medical devices and older people. His interests include using interpretative phenomenological methods to describe the psychosocial impact of medical technologies. He is the lead author of Chapter 10.

Address: Faculty of Engineering, University of Nottingham, Nottingham, NG7 2RD, U.K.

Heather Underwood is a Ph.D. Candidate in the ATLAS Institute at the University of Colorado Boulder. Her research focuses on the use of information and communication technologies for the developing world. She is the author of Chapter 12.

Address: University of Colorado Boulder, 1125 18th St., 320 UCB, Boulder, CO, 80309 U.S.

Jayne Wallace is a Reader in Design at University of Dundee. Her research centres on co-creative empathic design practices in the creation of digital artifacts to support wellbeing and sense of self. She has been working for many years with people with dementia and their carers. She is a co-author of Chapter 9.

Address: University of Dundee, Dundee DD1 5HN, U.K.

CPSIA information can be obtained at www.ICGtesting.com
Printed in the USA
LVOW03s0051210514

386619LV00006B/55/P